RES
SPIRITUAL
SKEPTICISM
IN RECOVERY

MW01194146

RESOLVING
SPIRITUAL
SKEPTICISM
IN RECOVERY

PUTTING THE UNIVERSE
TO WORK FOR YOU

ANDREW G. PIERCE, MCAP

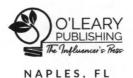

O'LEARY
PUBLISHING
The Influencer's Press

NAPLES, FL

Copyright © 2021 by Andrew G. Pierce
All rights reserved.

Published in the United States by
O'Leary Publishing
www.olearypublishing.com

The views, information, or opinions expressed in this book are solely those of the authors involved and do not necessarily represent those of O'Leary Publishing, LLC.

The author has made every effort possible to ensure the accuracy of the information presented in this book. However, the information herein is sold without warranty, either expressed or implied. Neither the author, publisher, nor any dealer or distributor of this book will be held liable for any damages caused either directly or indirectly by the instructions or information contained in this book. You are encouraged to seek professional advice before taking any action mentioned herein.

All rights reserved. No part of this book may be reproduced or transmitted in any form by any means, electronic, mechanical, photocopy, recording, or other without the prior and express written permission of the author, except for brief cited quotes. For information on getting permission for reprints and excerpts, contact: O'Leary Publishing.

ISBN: 978-1-952491-19-1 (print)
ISBN: 978-1-952491-20-7 (ebook)
Library of Congress Control Number: 2021910668

Editing by Heather Davis Desrocher
Proofreading by Kat Langenheim
Cover and interior design by Jessica Angerstein

Printed in the United States of America

This book is dedicated to
the circumstances and people
who caused so much pain that
I had to do something about it.

IMPORTANT!

This book has a vault of
digital resources that are essential
to the experience of this book.
To unlock them for
your personal use please visit:

www.andrewgpierce.com/book-links

CONTENTS

The most valuable gifts
are often wrapped
in the most beautiful pain.

PREFACE

I can't count the number of times I attended a 12-Step meeting early in my recovery where it wasn't long before someone began spouting off things like how great God is, or how their lives have changed completely since they came to *know God*, or that they know that God is doing this or that in their lives, or my least favorite, "God spoke to me this morning, and said _____ . . .", etc. At these moments I would develop a reflexive disdain for both the individual and their message as they spoke of things about which I was unable to relate. At times I would block out anything they said thereafter.

Why would I be experiencing this strong reaction? I would ask myself. I intuitively knew that those with any devoutness in their spiritual beliefs enjoy a quality of recovery that I could not relate to. If I were honest, I would have to say that I was always somewhat jealous of these people because *they had something that I wanted.*

In recovery, we learn to seek out *those who have what we want* recovery-wise — the idea being that someone with a great quality of recovery is someone we would likely benefit from knowing, relating to, and emulating so that we, too, could have what they had — that *thing* we intuitively find to be compelling about their attitude or insights.

Perhaps one reason for my reflexive disdain in these circumstances was partly because this woo-hoo (*fingers mockingly flitting*

about) spiritual type of conversation was in stark contrast to everything shared in the meeting up to that point — content to which I
could relate, nearly verbatim, about others' experience, hope, and
how they changed. Why did these God-talking people's words turn
me into such a resentful state that I would end up dissociating with
the entire meeting?

Were I to apply some psychology to myself, I would probably
conclude that in these moments of anger I was engaged in projection — directing anger toward another person that was *really*
intended toward a part of myself that I found unacceptable. Of
course, the problem with projection is that when we are focused on
others, we are not focused on ourselves, and we impair our ability
to grow. It is easier to criticize others than to look at ourselves.

The 12 Steps of Alcoholics Anonymous have *Higher Power* written all over them, so what chance did I have at long-term recovery
if I could not identify with a core aspect of the recovery program
— a program demonstrably capable of working for tens of millions
of people?!

I never met anyone too dumb to get sober, but I have met many
people *too smart* to get sober. I know that being overly analytical can
undermine spiritual efforts. For me, the solution to this dilemma
lay in applying whatever intellect I could muster toward gaining a
deeper understanding of something about which I have always been
fascinated — physics. Physics is the science of explaining reality. Its
study, however, exposes limitations on our ability to discover, and
our ability to ask the right questions, which is more like philosophy.

As an armchair physicist fascinated by how things work,
I explored, over the course of a year or so, ideas that have only
become proven science within the past decade. These new ideas
resolved my inability to embrace the existence of a higher power.

Addiction is a stress-response — an external attempt to solve an internal problem. Spirituality and the benefits it affords provides relief from stress, making it a practical tool with which to resist relapse. It is an internal solution to an internal problem, which is why it is effective.

HOW THIS BOOK WORKS

This book is actually two books (so congratulations on getting a deal)!

Part I of this book is all about how addiction works, and how its pathology undermines our ability to plausibly consider — much less trust — a higher power. It is very densely written, and as such will provide new insights upon each reading as you internalize the material. Passages you were unable to relate during one reading may take on new meaning during another reading.

Part II systematically explores the science and physics behind the author's Unified Theory of Recovery (UTR) clinical model, which he uses in his practice, as well as its implications for our recovery experience. It is all about how up-to-the-second quantum physics works, and how fusing ancient Eastern philosophy with it provides the basis for our ability to adopt a spiritual perspective that overcomes the barriers imposed by addiction (as outlined in Part I). Those well-versed in addiction and recovery may choose to skip Part I entirely, to get to the science that enables us to resolve spiritual skepticism. Part II imparts understanding of how we may participate as co-gods in not only our recovery process, but in fulfilling our destiny.

Every chapter, whether in Part I or II, addresses three primary themes

Stage 1 Recovery—Relapse Prevention

Stage 2 Recovery—Regain Authenticity

Stage 3 Recovery—Developing the Capacity for Spirituality

EXPERTISE ON LOAN FROM—EVERYONE!

This book uses third-party material in the form of videos and documentaries. The subject matter experts responsible for said content possess credibility and knowledge that inform the UTR Model — thus the term "Unified." This content illustrates the concepts crucial to understanding UTR, tying in disciplines such as

Substance use disorder	Consciousness
Shame	Mindfulness/meditation
Low self-esteem	Family of origin theory
Evidence-based change theories (REBT, DBT, etc.)	Eastern and Western philosophies
Quantum field theory	Quantum mechanics
Psychoneuroimmunology	Relational dynamics
Emotional sobriety	

UTR unifies these disciplines for one purpose — accelerating the rate and depth of recovery from addictions.

The subject matter experts include Gabor Mate, Brené Brown, David Greene, Arvin Ashe, Jim Al-Khalili, Aaron Beck, Alan Berger, Don Miguel Ruiz, Earnie Larsen, Melodie Beattie, Tony Robbins, Russell Brand, Viktor Frankl, Eckhart Tolle, Mooji, and numerous others.

I combine the contributions of these masters of their respective fields with traditional recovery sources including AA (Alcoholics

Anonymous) reading materials and concepts, The ACA (Adult Children of Alcoholics & Dysfunctional Families) *Big Red Book*, and traditional clinical models to bear on patients' addiction and mental health issues.

My own experience and credentials as

1. A person in long-term recovery from addiction,

2. A graduate of the premier addiction counseling program in the world — the Hazelden Betty Ford Graduate School of Addiction Studies,

3. And a clinician with thousands of hours of clinical practice possessing the most advanced possible addiction certification available in the state of Florida, the MCAP (Master's Level Certified Addiction Professional)

have enabled me to connect the dots between all of these contributors' ideas, thus creating UTR.

When you encounter these icons:

 hyperlinks   videos

please view the corresponding content located in the companion media vault at:

www.andrewgpierce.com/book-links

The videos and hyperlinks are sequentially organized by chapter and number for intuitive access, with newer material building on previous content — so please view the companion material in the order presented.

Finally, it is worth pointing out that as much as anything, this book is an autobiography. It chronicles my own journey from the depths of addiction, through academic enlightenment, emotional enlightenment, and eventually to a place of spiritual enlightenment — the difference being that rather than being linearly laid out in an easy-to-follow progression, my journey was a winding and often complex and confusing path.

So think of this experience now as though you are enlisting the services of a mountain man in the early 1800s who has been across the plains and Rocky Mountains to the Pacific Coast, and is now meeting up with you in St. Louis to guide you through unfamiliar territory to your destination. But your destination, rather than being the mouth of the Columbia River in Oregon, is the edge of human understanding, where you will find your True Self and your identity as a member of the spiritual realm.

INTRODUCTION

One thing compelling me to write this book is the pain I witness while scrolling through social media groups dedicated to recovery in its various forms. People reaching out in anguish at their loved ones' ongoing, active addiction, or their own addictions — and the pain expressed as they unsuccessfully attempt to guarantee their behavior for one sole purpose — to become a safe person to love. Being a safe person to love is crucial because true love — authentic human connection — is the most wonderful experience we can have on earth. Addiction is a saccharine effort to occupy the space in our hearts that is intended for Love. When we succeed in recovery, love displaces addiction.

Those who have engaged in the material outlined in this book have experienced:

- Dramatic decrease in cravings in a remarkably brief time frame
- Increase in self-efficacy (belief that they can change AND also fully realize their potential)
- Unshakable belief in their future prospects (hope)
- Decrease in feelings of stress, anxiety, powerlessness, and depression
- Increase in confidence
- Decrease in shame

- Ability to meaningfully connect with others (love and be loved)
- Ability to shed their (former) identity as a drinker or drug user, etc.
- A sense of connection to a higher power in whom they could trust — along with all of the tangible and intangible benefits that such belief provides including peace of mind; fearlessness; comfort or revelry in the unknown; a deep sense of meaning and connection with the Universe; love on a spiritual level; and worthiness of love from others.

The Unified Theory of Recovery (UTR), the clinical track I've developed for those in recovery from addiction and who struggle with spirituality, enables patients to move into a high-quality state of recovery far faster than any program I've encountered. It is delivered utilizing evidence-based methods, and the enhanced rate and depth of recovery benefits patients as well as stakeholders in their lives.

This book provides much content from the UTR clinical track. The actual program is presently delivered by me in the form of weekend boot camps, virtual and in-person individual and group sessions. A clinical track manual for use in a clinical setting is available, along with workbooks. Online subscription content is also available at www.andrewgpierce.com.

The following is a glimpse of some conclusions we arrive at when we simultaneously apply the principles of recovery, quantum mechanics, quantum field theory, and consciousness:

The Universe is not static, but dynamic — possessing a consciousness.

The Universe is inherently benevolent — it wants good.

We ourselves, and everything around us, are part of the quantum field.

The quantum field is a two-way vehicle through which we commune with, and receive feedback from, the Universe.

All conscious beings are connected through the field.

The quantum field represents infinite possibilities at any given point in time.

We each author our own realities, either consciously or unconsciously, selecting from an infinite number of possibilities every moment.

The richness of an idealized (future) vision of ourselves and the world, along with the frequency, quality, and coherence of meditation practice, is directly proportional to the quality of feedback reciprocated by the Universe. In other words, the higher the quality and greater the specificity and emotional content of our intentions, the more specific and voluminous will be the Universe's response.

Our aspirations are future memories corresponding to an idealized state of being that exists in one potential reality, serving as a beacon toward which we may direct our energies.

The Universe wants us to be happy. It wants us to walk in a reality akin to our own version or definition of 'Heaven on Earth' where gratitude is the predominant emotion, and in which our potential is fully realized.

Living in our most-authentic state in the present affords us the best opportunity to realize the reality in which we aspire to live — compressing the time between now and then.

One of the beauties of UTR as a change model is that it does not require one to discard traditional conceptions of a higher power for those already comfortable with a particular brand of spirituality. The quantum fields, which will be described in Part II of this book, serve as the mechanism by which any traditional God may operate. We may insert *any* higher power into this system without contradicting science, nor whatever deity may be running the show.

UTR practitioners possess dual citizenship in both the physical and immaterial worlds. We differentiate ourselves as both thinkers and conscious observers of our thoughts, bringing to bear the full potential of the quantum field into our daily existence.

By the end of this book, you will understand that the UTR clinical model is *not* a classical linear cause-and-effect Newtonian model like most change models. With UTR, creating change is more like switching the stations on a TV with infinite channels, each corresponding to a possible future or timeline. Each "channel" is a lifepath — one of which contains our idealized self and reality. Incremental lateral moves are set into motion by conscious intentionality, requiring *much* less effort than traditional change because the Universe does all of the heavy lifting.

This book will demonstrate that:

1. Your past has nothing to do with your future.

2. There is a benevolent higher power that "wants" above all for you to fully realize your potential as a human being.

3. The mechanism by which we realize our full potential is the quantum field.

**Be prepared to be transformed
as you internalize this material.**

ABSTINENCE IS NOT THE ENDGAME

Many people incorrectly believe that the opposite of addiction is abstinence. And while it's true that abstinence from substances (I will use *substances* interchangeably for both substance and behavioral addictions) does, in itself, fix many life problems, it is not the end game. When an angry alcoholic puts the cork in the bottle, they just go from being a drunken asshole to an asshole. Without doing the work necessary to address the underlying factors behind a person's desire to self-medicate, the likelihood of relapse is far greater than if they go about engaging in a full recovery process.

What abstinence *does* accomplish is that it:

- provides accurate access to our emotions that, in turn,
- creates the circumstances whereby talk therapy can be effective that, in turn,
- allows patients to make necessary gains in self-awareness (the ability to think about what we're thinking about),
- engenders emotional intelligence (the ability to apply gained insights strategically in real time),
- enables accurate empathy with others,
- enhances our ability to boost self-esteem,
- allows for conscious selection of values,
- enables the ability to accurately self-assess,
- facilitates our ability to regain authenticity,
- provides access to our conscience and gut instincts — possibly for the first time in decades, and
- fosters our ability to identify, establish, and maintain healthy boundaries, among other gifts,

- enables parts of the brain physiologically damaged by chronic use to heal over the course of 18-24 months, restoring "normal" processing and decision-making, and
- empowers us to guarantee our behavior.

Abstinence is merely the portal through which we become able to gain access to what we REALLY want in life — the capacity to realize our potential, to love, and to be loved, which is the most wonderful experience we can have here on earth.

It is my experience that *lack* of love is one thing those in addiction attempt to compensate for in their lives. Lack of love, or *fear* of lack of love (abandonment) is a significant driver behind addiction for most afflicted with the disease.

Love *only* resides within the context of healthy relationships. Healthy relationships can *only* occur when we have accurate access to our emotions and perceptions (in abstinence). **When we become a safe person to love, the right people will have no choice but to love us.**

HOW TRADITIONAL RECOVERY WORKS

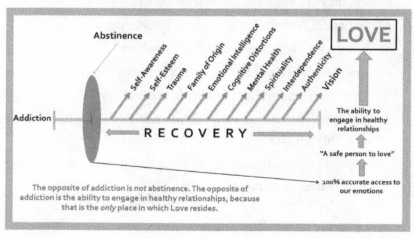

CRUCIAL PROBLEMS RESOLVED

This book addresses three main problems faced by most of us with addictions.

The first problem addressed is spiritual skepticism. As a fellow traveler in recovery, I *knew* that there were benefits to adopting a spiritual perspective, but for many valid reasons I was unable or unwilling. The work and research I undertook to find a solution to this problem is what this book is all about. This book gives you all the goods without all of the work.

Another area that those in recovery struggle with is self-esteem. The disease of addiction is often a disease of not feeling good enough. In my case crippling shame negatively impacted every major decision I made from childhood through adulthood: relationship choices, career choices, life choices such as marriage (that I didn't really want), finances, and how I was perceived by others. This shame made me vulnerable to manipulation and victimization. It also undermined my ability to function at the level I knew I was capable of reaching. When my reality exceeded that which I unconsciously felt I deserved, I would self-sabotage, either by inaction or by some other means. Does any of this sound familiar?

Now, I can see how low self-esteem affected all areas of my life. Only after seeing and addressing it was I able to change my life. Self-awareness of these tendencies is critical if we are to effect lasting change.

The third problem faced by many of us in recovery is low self-efficacy — disbelief in our ability to change. A cursory understanding of quantum mechanics and its implications enables us to have belief in a future totally unrelated to our past, resolving this issue.

Reviewing, internalizing, and applying the material in this book will unlock hope, excitement for the future, peace of mind in the present, and gratitude for the past.

Recovery is about *doing* and *being*. Thinking, of course, comes first. Anything we have done or become was first a thought. Life's natural progression is to go from *thinking* to *doing* to *being*. Take driving a car, for example. Perhaps you remember the first time you drove a car. You get in, check the mirrors, push down the brake, make sure it's in Park. You start it up, check around you for obstacles, take your foot off the brake, and check the clearance of the other cars next to you as you back out and turn the wheel or come to a stop, etc.

Nowadays we **are** *drivers*. We hop in, sandwich and drink in hand, not even thinking about all that driving involves because over time we went through the process from *thinking* to *doing* to *being* (a driver).

Traditional recovery methods are much the same. We *learn* about:

- the disease
- coping skills/tools
- relapse-prevention insights and attitudes
- dealing with past traumas
- how to maintain our emotional center

Through *practice* over time, we internalize what we've learned as our brain and body heal. It becomes second-nature; and before long we *identify* as people in long-term recovery.

The meditative aspect of UTR accelerates this process, moving us from Thinking to Being. The Doing part of the process — meditation — provides a shortcut to Being (more on that later.)

THE UNIFIED THEORY OF RECOVERY IS BORN

A lecture by Dr. Joe Dispenza entitled, *You Are the Placebo,* provides a glimpse of his change model, aspects of which inform UTR. The aspirational profile of those in his audience (entrepreneurs) makes it relevant for those of us who aspire to fulfill our potential. It was this lecture that prompted me to research his work, and in the process come up with UTR. I realized his ideas had applications for those recovering from addiction and related pathologies.

 0.1

Dispenza's books were inspired by a process he developed for implementing *physical* change in the bodies of those stricken with physiological maladies for which conventional medicine had no answers, particularly neural damage. He had a spinal injury from which he was told he would not recover. He was inspired by the placebo effect whereby a group of individuals who *believe* they are receiving a treatment being tested (but who in reality are not) experience the benefits of the treatment. The placebo effect is a very real phenomenon. All clinical trials are required to include placebo groups to test the efficacy of their proposed drug. The placebo effect may account for between 15-72 percent efficacy in relation to the group receiving the drug or treatment being tested, which is remarkable. The following link provides an example:

 0.2

Dispenza's methods leverage the placebo effect as well as other insights to favorably impact numerous physiological maladies — among them spinal injuries (including his own), cancers, immune-related deficiencies, etc.

Being a natural skeptic, I researched as much about Dispenza's work as I could. I concluded that his methods would be more than sufficient for treating addiction. After all, I don't need to repair anyone's spinal cord or cure cancer. While listening to one of his audiobooks, I began thinking about *how* I could apply the principles toward an addiction patient. The material fit remarkably well, and UTR was conceived.

HOW RECOVERY WORKS IN STAGES

One of the best overall summaries of what healthy recovery looks like comes from the primary text of Adult Children of Alcoholics & Dysfunctional Families (ACA) — the *Big Red Book*. This perspective of recovery touches not only on addiction, but also on the underlying issues that often both precede and accompany the disease. Many who enter ACA concurrently attend other 12-Step mutual support groups that address primary substance or behavioral addictions, otherwise known as Stage One recovery.

Stage One recovery involves stabilizing an individual from the immediate ravages of addiction so that they are able to abstain from engaging in addictive behaviors such as drinking alcohol, using drugs, gambling, spending compulsively, etc. This is often accomplished in mutual support groups, treatment centers, by engagement with an addiction therapist, or by some combination thereof. In a residential treatment setting the severity of patients' primary addiction necessitates all available resources be directed at stabilization. Invariably, patients are recommended to "step down" to a lower level of care after a residential treatment episode because we know that abstinence in itself is insufficient to maintain long-term sobriety and recovery. Stage Two work is usually added at these lower levels of care.

Since there are many excellent books and programs tailored to Stage One recovery, it is not the primary focus of this book; however, all of the material in this book is immediately beneficial to those engaged in Stage One of their process.

Stage Two recovery involves identifying and resolving the pain that addiction purports to medicate. So much of what makes an addict an addict has less to do with drugs and alcohol, and more to do with pain — after all, drugs medicate pain. That pain is what Stage Two recovery is designed to address. Dr. Gabor Mate' defines addiction as the effort to solve an internal problem by external means. Stage Two work can take time with traditional methods — the internal motivation of the patient and quality of therapist being primary determinants. This work is often accomplished through interaction with a therapist, and addresses factors not resolved in a treatment center setting because, again, stabilization takes up so much of the bandwidth in a residential episode.

Goals of Stage Two recovery work include regaining our authenticity (reconnecting with our True Self); addressing unresolved hurts, losses, and traumas; identifying, establishing, and maintaining healthy boundaries; and working through issues addicts use drinking or drug use to solve (or avoid).

Stage Three recovery is the phase in the recovery process where spirituality is introduced. The quality of our Stage Two recovery work determines the ease with which we are able to engage in Stage Three recovery. In Stage Three work, we refine our relationship with ourselves. In Stage Three, we have already undergone the process of regaining our authenticity, or have regained access to our True Self, and have gained experience in asserting our true selves in real-world situations.

The ACA *Big Red Book* beautifully illustrates the nature of Stage Three recovery and its importance to spirituality when it states:

> " . . . *It usually becomes easier to realize a loving relationship with our Higher Power once we have done most of our Stage Two recovery work. This is because* **the False Self or ego cannot experientially relate to or know God,** *and* **the only part of us that can do this is our True Self,** *which we come to know in our Stage Two work.* **While the False Self may at best try to intellectualize a relationship with God, our True Self does it from its heart, with fewer words needed."** *(emphasis added)*

Stage Three recovery involves refining our relationship with our True Self and Higher Power experientially — *that* is the key word here — *experientially*.

We must do Stage Two work to *experience* **being** *who we are, authentically*. **Our degree of our understanding of and connection with our True Self dictates the extent of our ability to commune with any higher power.** Our quality of authenticity governs our rate of progress in recovery.

One may undergo the three phases of recovery linearly; however, most of us progress in all three stages simultaneously.

THE PRECIPITATING EVENT

In a clinical setting, I have often disclosed aspects of my background for the purpose of conveying to patients that *I have been where they have been*, despite the details being different. It is important for those with whom a therapist works to understand and believe that their therapist is able to accurately empathize with them. After all, it doesn't matter how good a clinician is if the patient doesn't believe that their therapist can relate to them.

Many of the self-descriptive anecdotes I share raise a few eyebrows — a fact that I find amusing at times. Many patients will usually reply, "Wow, I can't believe you did that." or "That doesn't seem like you." to which I point out that this is what the change process does for us. We can't expect long-term fundamental change as the same person we were. We literally have to become someone else if we are to expect different outcomes.

With that in mind, let's step back in time for a moment to April 26, 2014 — the last day of my life in active addiction — to see how my fundamental change began.

I woke up on top of the covers, which is unusual for me as it probably is for anyone. It was a Saturday. Coincidentally, it was my wife's birthday; and oddly, the bed was made, which was somewhat confusing as most people sleep underneath the covers — and even if they are sleeping on top of the covers the bed is not already made before they wake up.

I checked my watch, and it was about 10 a.m. I called out to see if my wife was there in the apartment, and when she wasn't, I figured maybe she'd gone to the store to get some groceries or something along those lines. So, I called her up to see what was going on, and when she answered I said, "Hey, what's going on?" to which she replied, "Don't you remember what happened last night?" (This is never a good question to be asked in these circumstances.) Puzzled, I said "No, not really." She went on to say, "Well, last night you told me about the girlfriend you've been seeing for the last eight months who's 'half my age and twice as good-looking,' and that you're leaving me for her."

She continued with something to the effect that she had spent the entire night on the phone vacillating between crying to my mother and trying to figure out what to do next, and that through that process they had secured me a bed at the Betty Ford Center in Rancho Mirage, CA, and, by the way, someone was going to be coming by around 2 o'clock in the afternoon, to pick me up. I don't remember the rest of the conversation, but being a committed part-ier, I did check my watch thinking, 'Well, it's 10 o'clock now . . . that gives me four hours before they take me away. It's ON.'

I went down to find my car, which I had done pretty much every morning since we'd moved to Sherman Oaks. This ritual was because I was usually blacked out by the time I got home each evening around 6:30 or 7 p.m. (My wife worked for the studios, and she was rarely home before 7 p.m. most days, so I usually had plenty of time after work to do whatever.) At the time, I had a fairly new, white BMW 335i with a Dinan Stage III kit, a red leather interior, 400+ HP at the rear wheels, etc. But I digress.

So, I found my car, hopped in, and reached back to grab the box full of coke (not the beverage) I usually had stashed behind the passenger seat. I cut out a few long lines, took a few hits off from my dugout one-hitter (pot), and headed off to Champ's in Burbank for my last hurrah. On my way to the bar, I noticed that the glass from the passenger side-view mirror was missing. I shrugged, thinking, 'Guess someone must've needed it more than I did.'

I drove up to the curb in front of my favorite watering hole (where my nickname was The Captain, as that was my drink, Captain & Diet), got out of the car, and angled off to the bar's entrance. I happened to glance back, and was horrified to see that the passenger side looked as though it had been in a huge accident — which obviously must have occurred the night before on my way home from wherever I was (I don't actually remember much of the two months leading up to this day, due to the 300 Xanax I had purchased from my dealer friend back in February). The car was in bad shape. The front right bumper was crunched in as though I'd hit a light pole. The front right quarter panel looked like crinkled aluminum foil. The front passenger door looked about the same, and the first part of the rear passenger door was indented in continuation of the front door's damage from whatever it was I had sideswiped. There were a few faint red and yellow streaks from something I'd hit — so I closely examined the damaged areas looking for hair, or blood, or both. It struck me as odd that on the ride over my alignment had not been affected, as the car drove perfectly from the apartment.

There was no blood or hair in any of the many sharp indentations. So thinking, no body, no crime, I went into the bar and proceeded to order my usual Captain and Diet, repeating as needed until approximately 1:30 p.m. when I presumably paid my bill, hopped back in the car, and drove home to be hauled off to the Betty Ford Center.

I don't remember the drive home (as usual), but obviously I made it, and on time. I don't remember walking into the apartment either, but I'm told that among other things, I grabbed my rock-climbing rope and locked myself in the bathroom verbalizing intent to hang myself (although in retrospect I'm fairly sure that was just for dramatic effect). I was also told that I tried jumping out of the third story window of the apartment but was stopped, and that a few picture frames were smashed during the ruckus. Whatever the case, I eventually settled down, got down to the guy's minivan, and off we went to Rancho Mirage. Supposedly, I slept most of the way and upon check-in I'm told the driver needed help getting me to the intake department where I was processed, and ultimately admitted into the detox unit.

That was April 26, 2014, and I haven't used drugs or drunk alcohol since.

Treatment was awesome, as one might expect when residing inside the bubble of a treatment center with tons of support and no day-to-day stressors inherent to life outside the facility. In fact, I don't think I've ever laughed so much in my life. But eventually I had to leave treatment.

There were many challenges in my early recovery. I initiated and lost a few primary relationships. I spent the first two years with relatively little support except periodic AA meetings, and I spent a lot of time in loneliness. I struggled with daily life and emotions while having little self-awareness with which to navigate them. I know what it's like to go from using to abstaining with no real program of recovery. I also suffered financial pain and uncertainty. To borrow a clinical term — it sucked.

HOW SERENDIPITY WORKS

About a year into my recovery, my buddy Tom suggested I go back to school to become a counselor. I laughed it off, having graduated from college some 25 years earlier. But, a few days later, out of the blue, an email from my alma mater treatment facility — The Betty Ford Center — came across my inbox touting their grad school program. So, figuring *What have I got to lose?* I applied to their graduate school, never really expecting they would be interested in me.

I was wrong.

After a rigorous admission process (I still have the reference letters and admission essay somewhere on my hard drive), I was accepted to the Hazelden Betty Ford Graduate School of Addiction Studies. I had to wait until I had two years of sobriety under my belt, because at that school, students do their clinical practicum concurrently with school, and they don't want those new to recovery working with patients. So, I still had a year to go before I could start.

Nonetheless, I had a renewed interest in life as I began envisioning all of the good I could do as a counselor. Not coincidentally, this is one of the experiences I draw upon when encouraging patients to envision a compelling future. Without it, one remains rudderless and despondent at the thought of a meaningless, stagnant life.

The compelling future I envisioned back then has become reality many times over. Remember, every good thing we have ever experienced originated as a thought. This will become important as we move forward.

The 12th Step of the 12-Step recovery model states, "Having had a spiritual awakening as the result of these steps, we tried to carry this message to other alcoholics, and to practice these principles in all our affairs." This book is somewhat autobiographical in that it outlines and details the *spiritual awakening* I experienced, the lack of which (spirituality) necessitated the advent of my own clinical model (UTR) designed for those suffering in recovery without the benefit of spirituality. Any suffering I now experience stems from my own unchecked habitual thoughts, not my circumstances.

Necessity is the mother of invention. Many worthy clinical models have come into being over the years — all out of necessity — UTR now taking its place among them. There are *many* ways to get and remain sober, and the right one is *whichever works*. Nothing else matters, as long as it works for the individual seeking relief. This is why a good addiction therapist is fluent in all modes of treatment, enabling them to select those that will best serve the patient.

HOW ADDICTION WORKS

— OR —

HOW SCREWED UP WE REALLY ARE

Popular self-help books are written for the general public. Over 10 percent of the population, however, is afflicted with addiction, and would not be able to relate to what a fully realized version of themselves would "be" like. It is impossible for those afflicted with addiction to imagine a world where every day is filled with gratitude and love. The principles laid out within most self-help books are just not accessible to those in early recovery or in addiction.

CHAPTER 1

HOW ADDICTION IS A DISEASE

When reading a self-help book, my mind is often thinking, *Wow, this is great; but, how could I tailor this material to be of benefit to someone who possesses the 'extra layer' of pathology addiction carries with it?*

Someone far more intelligent than I once said, "The beginning of understanding is the definition of terms."

The American Society of Addiction Medicine (ASAM) definition of addiction is as follows:

> *Addiction is a stress-induced, primary, chronic and relapsing brain disease of reward, memory, motivation, and related circuitry that alters motivational hierarchies such that addictive behaviors supplant healthy, self-care behaviors.*

One of the most accessible resources I have encountered on the etiology of addiction is a lecture by Dr. Kevin McCauley. He has a relatable way of explaining how addiction works.

While undergoing my practicum at Hazelden in Center City, MN, during "family week," this material was the first that family members were exposed to in the form of a documentary entitled, *Pleasure Unwoven*. It provides a succinct description of what is going on in their loved one's brains and explains their seemingly willfully bad behavior. It makes a strong case for the disease model of addiction that alleviates both the loved one and patient from misguided shame, enabling them to adopt a healthier perspective that "the problem is the problem" not the patient.

In his work, Dr. McCauley points out five primary contributors to faulty decision-making inherent to those in active addiction:

1. **Genetics** (approximately 40-60 percent of the contribution to one's potential vulnerability to acquiring a substance use disorder),
2. **Reward** (dopamine/salience to survival),
3. **Memory** (glutamate, locking in of dopamine-rich experiences for future reference: "triggers"),
4. **Stress** (environmental and self-imposed), and
5. **Choice** (executive function intended to mediate impulsivity).

Genetics account for between 40-60 percent of our potential vulnerability to addiction. The greatest physiological impact from a genetics perspective occurs in the mid-brain "reward" region of the brain from whence craving and drug-seeking impulses originate. This pre-corrupted data is passed along to the frontal cortex for processing with predictably questionable outcomes.

On a macro-level the brain is an organ, plain and simple. When one considers the complexities faced by the average person on a day-to-day basis — the decisions, their implications, and the cognitive ability we need to succeed at a sustainable level — we realize the brain truly is a wonder of nature.

As with *any* organ, however, the brain is subject to failure.

Chronic use of alcohol and drugs compromise the integrity of the delicate neural connections and related mechanisms whereby processing is accomplished. Despite this damage, thanks to neuro-plasticity (the remarkable ability to develop neural work-arounds), the brain may be able to *approximate* intended results; but, with chronic use the density, structure, and capacity of many areas of the brain become damaged to the extent that they no longer function properly. The good news is that with prolonged abstinence (18-24 months) the brain is able to repair itself.

HOW ADDICTION AND ADD ARE COUSINS

In addiction, one of the midbrain's genetic defects is a shortage of dopamine D2 receptors that may (or may not) have existed prior to patients' chronic substance use. An example of this scenario in action prior to addiction would be childhood ADD, which is exemplified by

- impulsivity,
- risk-taking,
- novelty-seeking,
- difficulty staying on-task,
- impaired follow-through,
- becoming easily bored or
- easily distracted,
- possessing enhanced natural curiosity,
- above-average intelligence,
- precociousness,

- inquisitiveness,
- unusually specific interests,
- creativity, and
- difficulty identifying and/or conforming to social norms.

One of the most noteworthy visuals in Dr. McCauley's presentation is below. He states, almost in passing, that what he sees when viewing the dopamine activity of those in addiction is the same thing he sees in scans of those afflicted with childhood and adult ADD — the basis for both being a shortage of dopamine D2 receptors.

 1.2

The illustration below contains Functional Magnetic Resonance Imaging (FMRI) scans. Each of the left-hand column's brains corresponds to those in the right-hand column. Each row shows the same brain; but, the left-hand column's images were taken prior to the subject's addiction to substances such as cocaine, methamphetamine, alcohol, and heroin. The pre-addiction images show much more dopamine receptor activity, as evidenced by the preponderance of yellow, orange, and red coloring in the midbrain.

The right-hand column shows addicted brain scans of the same brains *after* addiction to the various substances, but in the absence of said substances. The scans show greatly decreased dopamine receptor activity, as evidenced by the lack of yellow, orange, and blue coloring in the corresponding images.

The FMRI brain scans of children and adults with ADD are similar to those in the addicted brain column, varying by degree of the severity of their ADD, as compared with a non-ADD's brain scans. Those with dopamine-starved midbrains from ADD are not only more vulnerable to addiction physiologically, but also as a result of environmental feedback from an ADD's symptomatic behaviors.

DOPAMINE D2 RECEPTOR PAUCITY = ADD AND ADDICTION

DOPAMINE D2 RECEPTORS ARE LOWER IN ADDICTION

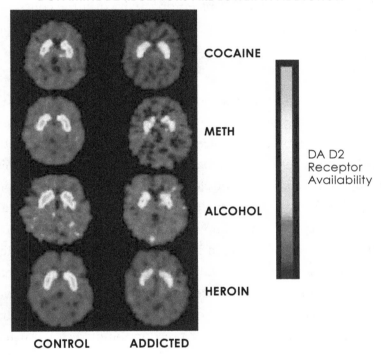

Within my practice, approximately 70-80 percent of those presenting for addiction therapy either had, or have, childhood or adult ADD. So, it would be negligent not to point out the importance of ADD in any discussion of addiction due to the high correlation between the brain's blueprint in those with ADD and those in chronic addiction.

With chronic substance use this condition only worsens over time, making early recovery challenging, as patients are even more restless, irritable, and discontented than they were prior to initiation of substance use.

The FMRI brain scan below shows the relatively rapid rate of decline of baseline dopamine receptor activity over the course of a year for someone using cocaine.

 1.3

Not surprisingly, it has been my experience that those who are or have been diagnosed with ADD have naturally gravitated toward cocaine as a substance of choice to the extent that in my practice it has become cliche'. This is because, under its effect, dopamine levels approximate something closer to that of a normal brain, providing relief from the emotional and mental suffering a shortage of dopamine receptor activity imposes on those afflicted with ADD.

The other side of that coin is that in early recovery, a patient may be mis-diagnosed with adult ADD due to symptomatic behavior of those whose dopamine receptor activity has been eroded with chronic use. As the brain heals over the course of a year or two, it will be easier to assess whether a prescription medication will be beneficial. The brain's dopamine activity may well restore itself in abstinence, negating the need for remedial medications.

COCAINE—D2 RECEPTOR AVAILABILITY OVER TIME

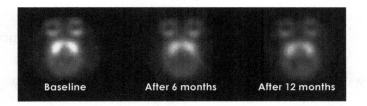

There are those who maintain that medicating children with stimulants to treat childhood ADD is a bad idea. This attitude is often informed by the view that it is simply *bad* to introduce chemicals into children for any reason whatsoever, unless perhaps the child is in an acute life-threatening situation. But most parents will acquiesce to the introduction of foreign substances (drugs) if their child is in the emergency room or hospital for the purposes of healing the child from an acute malady — even in overcoming cold or flu symptoms.

Another barrier to the introduction of stimulant medications for children with ADD is stigma. In such instances, parents are resistant to the idea of having their child take a drug because in doing so they would be admitting, de facto, that there was *something wrong* with their child which, by extension, could imply (in their minds, at least) that there is something wrong with *them* — both ideas they find unacceptable. These irrational beliefs result in the child not receiving scientifically-proven, safe relief.

Withholding stimulant medication in children with ADD serves up a one-two punch in that the symptomatic behaviors, particularly those that cause frustration in the adults around them — parents, teachers, and peers — create environmental factors — *feedback* — from family members in particular — that foment both shame and low self-esteem in the child. Ultimately, the child, when exposed to alcohol or recreational drugs for the first time, experiences *profound* relief, which potentially sets them up for future struggles with addiction, and a string of tumultuous relationships in adulthood. Shame and low self-esteem acquired from these dysfunctional dynamics will likely inform all of that individual's relationships and decisions well into their adult life until intervened upon, and resolved through either therapy or treatment.

In most cases, the child becomes a "people-pleaser" who represses their authenticity in favor of maintaining attachment to whomever will love them — and at any cost. That cost is often horrific. The slow, yet certain accumulation of resentment that is a by-product of this repressive dynamic eventually becomes an unlimited cesspool fueling depression, chronic physiological disease, and/or addiction until reconciled. Self-repression can also result in compulsive cutting, mental health problems, and even criminally deviant behaviors that could lead to incarceration.

Some develop resilience to adapt.

Dozens of peer-reviewed case studies over the last few decades demonstrate that medicating a paucity of dopamine D2 receptors (childhood ADD) in children, using stimulant medications, *decreases* their susceptibility to addiction in their adult years. One implication of this is that, although genetically originated contributors to vulnerability to addiction exist, environmental factors are *far* more influential.

Longitudinal MRI studies have shown that chronic exposure to addictive substances destroys dopamine D2 receptors. Symptomatic behaviors such as becoming easily bored, impulsivity, risk-taking, novelty-seeking, poor judgment, etc. manifest in addicts regardless of whether or not D2 receptor paucity preceded chronic substance use. Those with childhood or adult ADD simply have a head start.

SUMMARY

STAGE 1 RECOVERY — PREVENT RELAPSE

+ Addiction is a disease due to the fact that although symptomatic behaviors can be averted, cravings, in themselves, stem from mid-brain physiological anomalies and are not within the control of the addict.

+ Addiction and ADD are related due to their origin in dopamine paucity in the midbrain.

+ Those with untreated ADD are more vulnerable to addiction than the average person.

+ Treating childhood ADD with proper medication *decreases* the incidence of addiction among those diagnosed with ADD.

STAGE 2 RECOVERY — REGAIN AUTHENTICITY

+ Although addiction's symptomatic behaviors have moral implications (due to the defect being in the pleasure and reward center of the brain), the reality is that addiction is a disease in the same manner as diabetes — managed with proper treatment. This knowledge makes self-acceptance easier, as we realize our addictive behavior did not reflect our True Self.

+ Despite symptomatic, shameful behaviors, those with addiction should be treated as patients, and not as criminals. Punishing addicts is counterproductive to recovery in every way.

STAGE 3 RECOVERY — ENHANCE SPIRITUAL CAPACITY

+ Proper treatment allows us to guarantee our behavior. This, in turn, decreases our shame, and self-esteem improves. As such, we feel more worthy of, and less resistant to, connection with a higher power.

CHAPTER 2

HOW THE BRAIN WORKS

HOW SUBSTANCE USE DAMAGES THE BRAIN, AND VICE VERSA

Addiction is marked by consistently faulty decision-making, and recovery is evidenced by making consistently better decisions. Since the brain is an organ, and the fountainhead of addiction lies in the brain, it is useful to understand how the parts of the brain are adversely affected by addiction, and how that damage then perpetuates it. In addition to the midbrain, three distinct parts of the frontal cortex — the executive branch of the brain — are impacted by substance use. The science and psychology associated with this damage is both fascinating and scary.

THE ORBITOFRONTAL CORTEX

The orbitofrontal cortex (OFC) is responsible for, among other things, assigning relative value to things and experiences in our environment, guiding our decision making.

Back before Functional Magnetic Resonance Imaging (FMRI) made it possible to measure real-time brain activity, researchers used to have to sit around and wait for someone to have a stroke in a particular part of their brain and then watch their behavior to gain insight as to the practical function(s) of various parts of the brain. It was observed over the years that people who had a stroke in their orbitofrontal cortex had difficulty assigning relative value to things in their environment. For example, someone who had a stroke in their OFC could be shown three items such as a laptop computer, a car, and a house. While the patient could name the items and describe their function, he or she could not value them accurately in relation to each other.

You may say, "So what? They may not do very well playing *"The Price Is Right*?!" Well, it turns out this *is* a big deal, because these patients' lives eventually fall apart as they could no longer ascribe appropriate salience to money, their jobs, their spouses, children, etc. These unfortunates lost the rudder by which they guide value-based decisions. Those with addicted loved ones have witnessed the symptomatic behaviors of damage to this area of the brain — the legal, emotional, physical, relational, and financial consequences.

THE ANTERIOR CINGULATE CORTEX

Another part of the brain that is damaged by substance use is the anterior cingulate cortex (ACC), which is responsible for, among other things, helping us self-assess by picking up on and interpreting social cues — the non-verbal communication that tells us *how we're doing* socially. This is important in navigating subtle social situations in the workplace and in our personal lives. Individuals with addiction-based damage to this part of the brain tend to be blind to body language. They may not be able to sense, for example, that a conversation has run its course as the other person in the conversation is clearly disengaging. They are also blind to social norms, resulting in a tendency to stick out socially.

A damaged ACC is also responsible for an addicted person being the last to realize they have a problem (although it may be obvious to everyone around them). Ironically, those with damaged ACCs are perfectly able to assess the implications of others' decisions and actions which, if you stop to think about it, is at least one reason why AA and the interdependence of fellowship "works." Such mutual support groups are literally a bunch of people with damaged ACCs leveraging each other's ACCs to their mutual benefit.

Left to their own devices, a person in early recovery from a substance use disorder may with good intention think to himself, *I think I'm going to go to Key West this weekend by myself, chill on the beach watching people go by, and sip a Diet Coke.* Now, anyone who has ever been to Key West (and remembers it) knows that adults do not go there to sit on the beach and drink soft drinks. They go there to party. Hard. It is not a sober-friendly destination. So, considering the dynamics associated with such an environment, only a fool would expect a favorable outcome, alone, in early recovery.

If I voiced my Key West idea in the company of another person in recovery, regardless of the condition of *their* ACC, they would look at me like I was an idiot, and say, "That is the stupidest idea I have ever heard. Why don't we do something around here, or at least if you are going to go, bring your sober posse with you to keep each other accountable?"

That is what fellowship in mutual support groups is all about. Our ability to self-assess is impaired, but our ability to assess others is perfectly clear, as is theirs toward us. In a mutual support setting, we essentially borrow someone else's ACC, resulting in far better decisions than were we left to our own devices. This is one of many reasons why interdependence with others in recovery is so crucial as opposed to either surrounding ourselves with old (using) friends or isolating. I like the saying, "An alcoholic in isolation is in terrible company."

The good news is that the brain heals itself with total abstinence from substances over the course of approximately 18-24 months, which among other reasons is why recovery becomes incrementally easier as each day passes.

For the record, I went to Key West with my wife a few months ago with the option to stay there overnight. Even I was getting a little squirrely before long, and after about three hours I was ready to get the hell outta Dodge.

And we did.

We watched the sunset as we drove the causeway back up north to Miami where we spent a wonderful evening — a beautiful drive.

THE INSULAR CORTEX

The third part of the frontal cortex, the Insular Cortex, is central to addiction's symptomatic behaviors. It is critical in the processing of emotion, decision-making, the ability to accurately empathize with others, self-awareness, craving, reward assessment under shifting risk conditions, and other crucial cognitive processing tasks. Many case studies have been done, particularly during the last decade since functional magnetic resonance imaging has come into being, allowing observation of live, functioning brains when exposed to varying environmental cues. Those observed in the past who had strokes in the insular region of their brains had some surprising addiction-related outcomes. For instance, there are anecdotes where a person with a smoking addiction would wake up in the hospital after a stroke and a buddy would offer them a cigarette on the low-down. The patient would look at them quizzically and say, "Are you kidding?! I don't smoke." In these patients, both the physical and mental nicotine addiction had completely vanished in these individuals. It was such instances that caused those in the addiction field to begin paying attention to this part of the brain.

Various studies since have revealed a number of notable findings relating to addiction's impact on the insular cortex:

Persistent substance use alters insular function and physiology (size and density).

The ability to connect the dots between symptomatic behaviors and negative consequences is impaired.

The insular cortex is an anatomical "integration hub" connecting sensory, emotional, motivational, and cognitive functions, and coordinates interplay between bodily feelings, decision making, and risk avoidance within the context of drug use.

Healthy insula promote emotional regulation and flexible behavior while a damaged insula promote persistent inflexible behavioral patterns motivated by (substance-related) drives and bodily feelings.

Damage to the insular cortex is associated with misplaced distrust of those who have demonstrated trustworthiness, and misplaced trust of those who have demonstrated willingness to betray them.

The insula is activated when emotions are observed in another human being such as pain or disgust, suggesting a role in accurate empathy — impaired with insular damage.

Those in active addiction steal from their grandparents, engage in infidelity, robbery, murder, betrayal and worse.

Eighty percent of those incarcerated or imprisoned are there for behaviors either directly related to substance use, or perpetrated to gain resources necessary to support their addictions. These statistics reflect, among other things, insular damage.

SYNAPTOGENESIS

One experiential aspect of addiction is *craving*, a phenomenon rooted in physiological anomaly within the midbrain and insular cortex. Substance use can cause an abnormal increase in some brain structures, particularly in neurons. The physical change to neurons is called synaptogenesis. Synaptogenesis is a process in which synaptic contacts form and mature. In the case of substance use, the synaptic neurons, or in the case of addiction, dendrites in the midbrain connecting the VTA and Nucleus Accumbens (the "pleasure circuit"), experience significant growth in thickness and density. This type of alteration occurs quickly, resulting in increased craving as neuronal superhighways are paved within *hours* of substance use, as evidenced in the illustration on the following page.

Decreased density and size of *some* brain structures such as the insular cortex result in abnormal cognitive processing activity. *Increase* in density of the reward circuitry's neural pathways only further complicates matters. As such, in early recovery the brain is pre-primed to relapse in both primary, and cross-addictions — anything to make use of the increased neural bandwidth afforded by synaptogenesis. This is one reason why fraternizing and developing new romantic relationships is discouraged in early recovery — sex being a strong pleasure/survival behavior. It is not because 12-Step members are puritanical.

SYNAPTOGENESIS

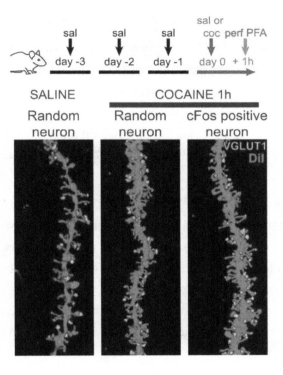

This critical early recovery period represents an opportunity to get a handle on what nonsexual and non-compulsive love is, as opposed to sprouting a sex addiction or perpetuating codependency, which is a fear-based, pathological need for emotional enmeshment — not Love.

That said, the good news is that studies also show that abstinence from all addictions over the course of 1½-2 years results in physical restoration of affected parts of the brain, making normal processing easier. As with all addiction-imposed brain damage, with few exceptions, the more time spent in abstinence, the better the long-term prospects for those in recovery.

SUMMARY

STAGE 1 RECOVERY — PREVENT RELAPSE

+ Understanding the physiology of addiction in the brain reduces shame as we realize that damage to the brain is behind our symptomatic behaviors. This decreases anxiety, reducing relapse potential.
+ Understanding the brain's ability to heal itself over the course of 18-24 months provides us hope for the future as craving depth and frequency subside.

STAGE 2 RECOVERY — REGAIN AUTHENTICITY

+ Understanding that in active addiction we are not our True Self, and that it is reversible via time and neuroplasticity, affords us the possibility to imagine a Self that differs from the addict we have become. Hope decreases stress.
+ In a state of decreased stress, we may become creative and imagine a life manifesting our True Self.

STAGE 3 RECOVERY — ENHANCE SPIRITUAL CAPACITY

+ The brain's neuroplasticity and ability to heal itself is truly miraculous. As it goes about this healing process, we become more receptive to the possibility that our healing will enable us to realize our full potential. In this way we remind others and ourselves how miraculous recovery, and our capacity to change, can be.
+ The brain's self-repair in abstinence from substances enables us to behave in a manner better-aligned with our values. Contemplating our innate values opens us to the possibility of a divine origin. Values such as growth, self-fulfillment, and love have basis in all spiritual doctrines.

CHAPTER 3

HOW OUR *OTHER* BRAIN WORKS

As discussed in the previous chapter, addiction-imposed brain damage causes an inability to self-assess or to empathize with others, and impairs our ability to connect the dots between our behaviors and consequences — even when *not* under influence.

But the brain is not the sole physiological factor in the disease of addiction. Interoceptive information is the sensory data the brain receives from the body. **The body has many times more channels going *into* the brain than coming out of the brain.** The information transmitted to the brain originates in the immune system, the gut, the bone marrow, the heart, and other structures. For instance, serotonin, the "feel good" hormone, primarily resides in the gut as opposed to the brain.

It is impossible to separate the emotional from the physiological aspects of our state of being. We are if nothing else, a circulating bag of chemicals. Our emotions are nothing more than electro-chemical interactions. The emotion of anger, for instance, is its own unique cocktail. So are longing, fear, compassion, affection, shame, happiness, and any other emotion we can imagine.

Over the last few decades, science has been able to accurately acquire data on how this works. In Dispenza's *You Are The Placebo* lecture (from the introduction), you may recall the fact that the chemical reaction comprising healthy anger is intended to last for approximately 90 seconds. Dispenza notes that anger exceeding any duration thereafter constitutes unhealthy anger, which is perpetuated by dysfunctional thought processes. If our goal in recovery is to manage stress, then it serves us to start thinking about what we're thinking about. For instance, what is it we *must* believe in order for our anger to last beyond 90 seconds? The same applies to any emotion — shame, in particular — that is perpetuated by deeply-ingrained pathological thought patterns originating in our family of origin, and reinforced by addiction.

In the following lecture Dr. Gabor Mate', a world-renowned subject matter expert on psychoneuroimmunology discusses how family dynamics during childhood impact our vulnerability to chronic illness, depression, and other mental health issues. The principles he lays out in the lecture apply to those in addiction.

 3.1

The same relational dynamics that set up Dr. Mate's patients for chronic illness set up a majority of those in addiction, and the codependents who love them, for significant strife until the dynamics are resolved. In his patients, and mine, the cumulative resentment of decades of "people-pleasing" is a pretense for chronic illnesses, depression and addiction. Resentment serves as rocket fuel for addiction or for potential relapse.

According to Mate', the physiological and emotional are not separate, nor even discreet from each other. In his work, Joe Dispenza acknowledges the importance of congruence between the mind and body in effective meditation. He notes that the body does not know the difference between a real experience and an imagined one (think pornography, right?).

Tony Robbins leverages physiology in his seminars via loud music and heightened emotions through movement to cement change.

HOW GUT INSTINCTS WORK

The *gut*, the source of gut-instincts, plays a role in both addiction and recovery. The gut contains billions of neurons identical to those in the brain, a number approximating that of a small animal such as a dog or cat. Both animals are adept at survival, and the gut is the apparatus we employ for that purpose.

We have relied on gut instincts for survival as a species for over a million years. Evolutionarily speaking, the gut precedes the prefrontal cortex, and necessarily so because were it not for accurate gut instincts as we were wandering about in the jungles or plains, we would not have survived as a species long enough to have developed a frontal cortex. To be more accurate, our gut was our *first brain*. Our gut instincts tell us whether people or situations are safe or not. Problems arise with our gut instincts when we engage in substance use.

ISOLATION IN ADDICTION

When we pollute our bodies with substances, *both* of our brains (the one in our head and the one in our gut) become impaired. The implications play out predictably. It is common knowledge that those with substance- use disorders tend to isolate. I distinctly recall when in active addiction, stating, "I hate people. They are nothing more than the orange cones in life to be navigated around."

From the standpoint of the gut's role in survival this should come as no surprise. Faced with an inability to accurately *read* people (or situations, for that matter) because the gut is polluted by substances, the safest thing to do is always to withdraw, or isolate. Isolation, for the most primitive reason imaginable — survival — becomes an obvious choice when driving blindly.

The first eight minutes of the following documentary provide a brief overview of the importance of the gut in the survival and evolution of our species.

3.2

An important distinction not made in the documentary, but which will become important later on, is that our gut is integral to regaining our True Self. **The gut is the primary sensory apparatus of our True Self.** We must become reacquainted with our True Self to develop a connection with a higher power, and abstinence is key to all of this.

Accurate access to our gut (instincts) is integral to Stage Two and Stage Three Recovery.

The Promises of AA indirectly mention a few benefits of this condition. For example, Promise 11 states, *"We will intuitively know how to handle situations which used to baffle us."* As we regain our gut instincts over time, we become more confident in our ability to read situations and others, resulting in the ability to relate better with them on a personal level. We also learn how to better relate to others in a work or business environment, resulting in the realization of another promise — Promise 10, which states, *"Fear of people and of economic insecurity will leave us."*

Restoring authenticity with an unpolluted gut enables others to read *us* more accurately, inspiring trust. Others sense, by subtle nonverbal cues, that we are trustworthy. Being perceived as trustworthy improves our economic prospects, as others crave authenticity in those with whom they associate, whether in their personal life, or in the business world.

SUMMARY

STAGE 1 RECOVERY — PREVENT RELAPSE

+ Gut instincts come online fairly quickly in abstinence from substances. As such, we become willing to rejoin the *human race,* learning to discern safe from unsafe people. At first, 12-Step meetings and therapeutic settings provide the safest forums in which to test out our newfound gut instincts — we learn to trust again.

+ As we gain experience trusting our gut instincts, we carry this out into the real world where we thrive in personal and business settings, decreasing financial stress, and opening us up to new romantic possibilities.

+ Successful connection with others decreases stress and relapse potential.

STAGE 2 RECOVERY — REGAIN AUTHENTICITY

+ Gut instincts are a buried remnant of our True Self that enabled us to survive as a species long before we developed a frontal cortex. When we were using alcohol and drugs, we polluted our "first brain" (gut) along with the one in our heads. Absence of any ability to discern who and what was safe brought us to the logical conclusion that the safest strategy for survival is to withdraw in isolation.

+ When others experience our True Self and our authenticity, they have no choice but to love us, and we are then able to develop self-love from both internal and external sources, expediting our recovery and confidence.

STAGE 3 RECOVERY — ENHANCE SPIRITUAL CAPACITY

+ Living in alignment with our gut instincts is an authentic act that enables successful, healthy relationships with safe people. As we have experiences where we are able to trust others, and to even experience true love, we may become more open to the possibility of trusting a higher power.

CHAPTER 4

HOW OUR THINKING PERPETUATES ADDICTION

Both genetic anomalies and addiction-imposed damage to the brain impact our thought processes in addiction, resulting in decisions that do not reflect our goals and values.

However, there are additional factors that play a significant role in our poor decision making.

If we use a computer analogy, the *software* with which we process this corrupt data is often rife with coding errors, compounding the likelihood of output (behavior) that does not align with our values and goals.

This state of affairs is not exclusive to those struggling with addiction. Mental health issues like codependency, anxiety, some forms of depression, phobias, obsessive-compulsive disorder (OCD), and dysfunctional relational dynamics, are all tied to these thinking errors. Brain damage is not required for this to occur.

And all of this processing takes 77 milliseconds.

Patients see me because they are consistently unable to get the outcomes they seek relationally, vocationally, financially, emotionally, vegetably, minerally, etc. They intend to start out their day in one way, and it almost always ends up in quite another.

No one wakes up one sunny morning, yawns, stretches, glances out the window, and says, "Gee, I think I'm going to go to treatment today!" To the contrary, the status quo has usually become unsustainable, and they realize the need to make a change. They need someone to look at their thinking, help them identify bad code, rip it out — and replace it with good code.

I liken their dilemma to a pilot who wishes to fly from Miami to Hawaii, yet who consistently ends up running out of fuel somewhere over the Indian Ocean. Clearly there is an error in either the hardware, or programming of their flight computer.

I firmly believe that those seeking my help possess everything they need between their ears to resolve their dilemma. They are simply missing information, and need someone whom they trust to act as a mirror to help them see blind spots in their understanding of themselves.

Given accurate information, they will be able to return to full functionality, and land in Hawaii consistently.

My job is to help patients get what they want. Together, we raise awareness of (formerly) unconscious beliefs and rules they picked up along the way that resulted in their continually ending up in the Indian Ocean. We determine whether these beliefs serve or undermine, and then we decide which to keep and which to shed.

Taking the computer analogy further, it is three hackers who consistently seem to install our bad code:

1. Family of Origin
2. Madison Avenue
3. Social Media

Absent self-awareness, these entities have had unfettered access to our belief systems, often to our detriment (see: any Instagram "reel" feed).

Faulty software increases stress. In fact, I would submit that 95-98 percent of our stress is self-imposed by erroneous processing of environmental factors — what they mean to us, and how we perceive them. When we are able to successfully reconcile thinking errors that cause us distress, we experience a more effortless and fulfilling recovery experience. The cognitive restructuring necessary to remedy self-imposed stress, anxiety, and depression is evidence-based, effective, and has been around for decades. If we do not understand how thinking errors affect our thinking and emotions, we are operating at a disadvantage.

The first step in addressing stress is to increase self-awareness, or the ability to think about what we are thinking about.

We assign meaning to circumstances, yielding emotion, followed by a choice as to how or whether to act — or not — which is informed by those prior factors. That choice impacts our circumstances, and the cycle repeats, ad infinitum. If I were to put this formula into a more formal format, it would read: Our circumstances, combined with our rules and beliefs, yield emotions, which then inform our decisions, which, in turn, affect our circumstances.

HOW WE MAKE CHOICES

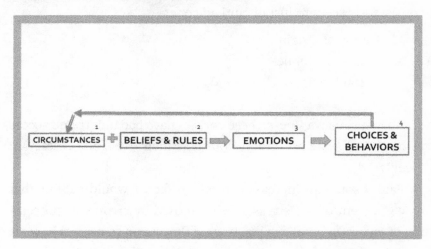

In the diagram, Box 1 represents our Circumstances or the *nouns* in our lives — they all boil down to people, places, and things. Box 2 comprises the conscious and unconscious Beliefs and Rules we possess about ourselves and our circumstances by which we assign *meaning* to whatever is in Box 1. The combination of our circumstances plus the meaning we assign them yields an emotion. So Box 3 is Emotions — either positive or negative and to varying degrees. Finally, Box 4 represents the choices and behaviors we engage in as a result of the previous three boxes that complete the circle by informing our circumstances.

This flowchart, properly applied, exposes beliefs held by those of us afflicted with addiction — beliefs that generate outcomes that differ from those of the so-called average person — particularly about who we are, what we are capable of, and what we deserve from life. I became emotional when writing that last sentence, because the things addicts *must* believe to be true about themselves in order to make the decisions they do, break my heart.

When I draw the above chart out on the ink board for patients, I ask them to rank them in order from that over which they believe they have the most control, to that over which they believe we have the least. Most patients will state that Choices and Behaviors are that over which we have the most control, usually followed by Emotions, then Circumstances, and finally Beliefs & Rules.

This is when I seize the opportunity to make a clear distinction between the 90 percent of so-called normal people and those of us fortunate enough to be blessed with addictive tendencies.

Let us say the average person's Circumstances are that they are 30 lbs. overweight. So, by my naive patient's logic they simply make a Choice (Box 4) to go to the gym and work out, therefore improving their Circumstances (Box 1) by lowering their weight, which places them in closer alignment with their Beliefs about what they should look like (Box 2), the ensuing Emotion being pride (Box 3), then of course reaffirms their Choice to continue going to the gym until they have accomplished their goal. Simple, right?

Given the fact that they are being asked this question within the context of a treatment center, I usually pivot to their substance-of-no-choice.

I say to them,

> Let us say your Circumstances are that your spouse has said they are going to leave you if you do not stop drinking, and for the sake of this argument you care whether they leave or not (because of your Rules and Beliefs). And by the way, they said this two years ago.
>
> Given your previous response, that Choice is that over which we have the greatest control, then the Emotions of shame and fear accompanying your spouse's threat (Circumstances) would

undoubtedly result in a Choice to stop drinking that would then positively affect your Circumstances (your spouse would stay), which aligns with your Beliefs and Rules about what a happy relationship should look like, thus yielding an Emotion of love and gratitude reinforcing that Choice to abstain from drinking, and so on.

Yet here we are having this conversation in a treatment center a year after they have left you.

Patients at this point usually default to Box 2, which, for those of us in addiction, is where the money is. (By the way, only crazy people simply go to the gym and accomplish their goals. Everyone knows that.)

We have the most control over our Beliefs and Rules. This is good news, because we are 100 percent in control over this aspect of our lives. No one can dictate these to us without our permission. It's just that no one told us.

The box over which we have the *least* control is Emotion, which is reflexive.

Addictive behaviors are *always* predicated upon uncomfortable Emotions that result from the Beliefs and Rules with which we assign meaning to our circumstances.

Addiction is, at its heart, a stress reaction. Our #1 job as a person in recovery is to be as non-reactive as possible to people, circumstances, and environmental factors (nouns).

Emotional self-regulation requires self-awareness. We must bring the unconscious to a conscious level. Only then are we able to *decide* which rules, beliefs, and values serve us and which to shed.

One tool I recommend patients use in order to gain insight as to Beliefs and Rules that cause them distress is to catch themselves being upset at a particular Circumstance, and then ask (and answer) the question, "What would I *have* to believe in order to feel this way?"

There may be far more than one response to this question. The idea is to get all of them, if possible. (More on this later.) But a good therapist acts as a mirror to patients to help them become aware of blind spots they never realized existed. Most people, when given enough insight about themselves, are able to effect the changes they desire. Actually, it could be no other way, because no one can change anyone but themselves.

Many, not just those in addiction, go through life oblivious to the Beliefs and Rules driving their behavior. They are proverbial leaves in the stream of life, obliviously bouncing off their environment with little understanding of who they are, or what they want in life. Their programming was installed by their parents as children, by Madison Avenue marketing whizzes as their little heads full of mush developed, and by any number of others wishing to impose their agenda on the unwitting oblivion. That's not living — it's existing.

Those of us fortunate enough to have been forced into some sort of therapeutic environment are at a huge advantage over those who have never had to self-evaluate. Again, the job of a therapist is to serve as a mirror for the purpose of pointing out blind spots in patients' self-understanding. The insights gained from a quality therapeutic relationship include:

- happiness,
- self-fulfillment,
- realization of potential,

- self-efficacy,
- shedding of fears,
- improved personal and professional relational dynamics,
- self-esteem,
- confidence,
- human connection,
- spiritual connection,
- reconnection with our True Self,
- and others too numerous to list.

The true scope of our influence does not exceed ourselves. The world and people in it are going to go about world-ing and people-ing, regardless of our efforts to control or change it. If we are not vigilant, environmental factors can undermine our peace of mind. It is not only the content of our thoughts, however, that serve as a source of distress. Distortions in the *logical structure* upon which we attach environmental factors, influences the meaning we assign them. More often than not, this logical framework is horrendously corrupt, leading to unnecessary self-imposed stress.

In the next chapter we will identify a number of opportunities to decrease relapse potential, improve our ability to regain our authenticity and self-regard, and to enhance our spiritual capacity.

SUMMARY

STAGE 1 RECOVERY — PREVENT RELAPSE

+ Understanding our unconscious beliefs and values affords us hope that we can, in fact, shape our future. With this new-found understanding comes hope for change on our terms. Hope decreases stress and relapse potential.

+ When we gain control over our beliefs and values, and see the impact of this on our lives, confidence replaces hopelessness and shame. Less shame means less fuel for addiction and relapse.

STAGE 2 RECOVERY — REGAIN AUTHENTICITY

+ Our beliefs and values were installed over the years, first by family members in early childhood (often by dysfunctional parents), and then by professional marketers, and social media. These unexamined beliefs told us what and who we had to be in order to be lovable. Consciously identifying these beliefs so we can be our True Selves is crucial for those expecting long-term change from addiction to recovery.

+ As we regain conscious awareness of factors influencing the meaning we assign to our circumstances, we regain control of our emotions, and thus our behaviors. When we are able to act in a manner aligned with our True Selves, self-esteem skyrockets.

STAGE 3 RECOVERY — ENHANCE SPIRITUAL CAPACITY

+ When we are able to see that perhaps our past experiences served a necessary purpose, the idea of a unique Universal plan becomes more plausible.

+ We may find the beliefs and values of our True Self intuitively resonate with spiritual paradigms we identified with prior to the genesis of our False Self.

CHAPTER 5

HOW OUR THINKING DOES NOT WORK

I THINK, THEREFORE I AM WRONG

Once we develop some self-awareness, we can begin identifying those rules and beliefs that are causing us to run out of fuel over the Indian Ocean. A tremendous number of mental health issues may be successfully resolved by our ability to identify and resolve *bad code* in our subconscious thinking. Crippling anxieties, depression, relationship struggles, shame, OCD, etc. have all been dealt with simply by the patient becoming aware of the presence of some (or many) of the seventeen most common *cognitive distortions*, as they are called in psychology work.

The reason for identifying and resolving these thinking errors in ourselves is that they are usually a source of stress — and totally unnecessary. Since addiction is perceived as an external "solution" intended to relieve emotional distress we *must* expose and root out these cognitive distortions. The result is a much more Zen, resilient, version of ourselves.

We already have everything we need right between our ears to make changes such as shedding addiction. Once we identify the thinking errors that are causing us distress, we are able to integrate new "code" into our mental calculus resulting in better decisions and outcomes. The resulting decrease in frequency and intensity of negative emotions reduces fuel for the desire to self-medicate.

In 1975, Aaron Beck took it upon himself to compile a list of the 17 most egregious offenders — cognitive distortions — to which no one is completely exempt. They are the focus of cognitive restructuring undergone in some form or another in most therapeutic settings. A person just entering into a therapeutic relationship usually looks something like this:

HOW MINIMAL SELF-AWARENESS WORKS

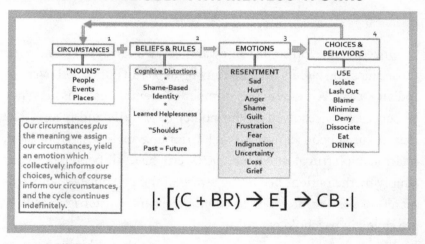

These 17 thinking errors fit into Box 2 — Beliefs & Rules — and their unconscious application to Circumstances negatively informs our emotions and decisions about what we do and say — or not. In tennis or baseball terms, these are all "unforced errors," as they are 100 percent within our capacity to identify and correct, with practice.

As you go through the following thinking errors, identify how strongly you relate with each distortion on a scale of 1-10. It may be easier to identify them in others than in yourself. If you have a significant other, it may be useful to ask them to rank their perception of the extent (if any) to which they apply to you.

1. ALL-OR-NOTHING THINKING

Also known as "Black-and-White Thinking," this distortion manifests as an inability or unwillingness to see things in shades of gray. Those with this perspective see things in terms of extremes — something is either fantastic or awful. You believe you or others are either perfect or suck. Others will either be in your life, or out of it, with no varying *degrees of engagement.*

It is easy to see why this cognitive distortion could be an impediment to one's peace of mind, particularly when on the receiving end of a relationship with such an individual. All-or-nothing people have a pattern of ending relationships abruptly, with little or no warning, as those in their lives inevitably fall short of their rigid expectations. This makes them unsafe to love, as evidenced by the number of people who they have alienated out of their lives over the years.

Those with all-or-nothing thinking say, and believe, things like, "If you're in second place, you're the No.1 loser." All or nothing thinking is often inherited through judgmental parents at an early age — parents whose own parents and grandparents likely were as well.

It is common among narcissists who feel compelled to present an image of perfection toward those with whom they are in a relationship. Narcissists prefer relationships with people with shame-based personalities such as those in addictions due to their ability to easily manipulate them with guilt and shame.

Since the world, and people in it, will never be perfect, those with polarized thinking cause themselves and everyone around them strife.

2. OVERGENERALIZING

This distortion takes one instance or example and generalizes it to an overall pattern, but with no basis for doing so. A student with this distortion may receive a marginal grade on a test and conclude that they are stupid and a failure. This type of thinking error leads to overly negative thoughts about ourselves and our environment based upon only one or two experiences.

Consider a door-to-door salesperson who gets out of their car first thing in the morning and knocks on someone's door only to be verbally assaulted by the occupant for interrupting their breakfast. This salesperson could easily think to themselves, "Ugh, I can see what kind of day *this* is going to be." which undermines the quality of their efforts for the remainder of the day as that one negative experience festers. Of course, the opposite could happen with the salesperson making a huge sale the first door-knocking of the day, and then overgeneralizing that experience to their *benefit*, bolstering their confidence and presentation with a *positive* outcome. But most people afflicted with chronic addictions tend to default to negative interpretations of singular events resulting in unnecessary distress.

3. MENTAL FILTER

The mental filter distortion focuses on a single negative piece of information, and filters out all positive ones. This occurs, for instance, when a partner in a romantic relationship dwells on a single negative comment made by the other partner, and then views the relationship as hopelessly lost despite years of positive comments and experiences.

The mental filter distortion fosters a pessimistic view by focusing only on the negative.

Another example is an individual undergoing an annual review by their employer, receiving top marks in all areas of their job performance but one, *opportunity for growth*. Someone with a mental filter distortion will ignore the positive feedback and become fixated on the *opportunity for growth* part of the overall message to their detriment.

This filter is prevalent in shame-based individuals such as those in or recovering from addiction who internalize feedback that resonates with their negative self-image. This is because negative feedback reaffirms what they already believe to be true about themselves — that they are unworthy of positive regard.

4. DISQUALIFYING THE POSITIVE

This distortion acknowledges positive experiences and feedback, but rejects them instead of embracing them. A person who receives a positive review at work rejects the idea that they are a competent employee, attributing the positive review to political correctness, or to their boss being a wimp and not wanting to talk about their *real* performance problems. A minority member with this distortion who gets a new job or promotion might attribute the accomplishment to race-weighted quotas as opposed to the employer thinking she is highly competent or qualified. This distortion perpetuates negative thought patterns in the face of strong evidence to the contrary.

5. JUMPING TO CONCLUSIONS — MIND READING

This distortion is the inaccurate belief that we *know* what another person is thinking. Of course, we may have an *idea* of what other people are thinking; but, this distortion refers to negative interpretations that we reflexively jump to. Seeing a stranger with a negative expression and jumping to the conclusion that they are thinking something judgmental about you would be an example of this distortion. Reflexively flipping off your grandmother who beeped her horn at you, because you thought it was someone beeping at you for another reason, might be another example.

I see mind-reading when working with couples who have been together for a long time. They become so familiar that they begin assigning negative meaning to non-verbal cues in the absence of data points, often coming to inaccurate conclusions to their mutual detriment.

Of course, when one of the partners is recovering from addiction, many of their partner's interpretations are expected to be negative, resulting in emotions such as rejection, animosity, and fear, which could lead to relapse or misguided dissolution of the relationship.

6. JUMPING TO CONCLUSIONS — FORTUNE TELLING

A sister distortion to mind reading, fortune telling, is making predictions based on little to no evidence, and then holding them as gospel truth. One example is a young, single woman predicting that she will *never* find love or have a committed and happy relationship, based solely on the fact that she has not found one *yet*. There is simply no way for her to *know* how her life will turn out; but, she views and experiences this prediction as fact rather than one of several possible outcomes.

People in addiction tend to predict the worst, based on past experiences. Stockbrokers are required to print, "Past performance does not guarantee future results" on any prospectus. Fortune Telling can undermine a person's recovery efforts by virtue of the belief that they are destined to a finite range of possibilities moving forward — that change is impossible. They falsely believe that past performance does guarantee future results. The corresponding feelings of hopelessness can foster relapse.

7. MAGNIFYING—CATASTROPHIZING

This distortion involves exaggerating the meaning, importance, or likelihood of our circumstances. A person in recovery who is generally solid but has a relapse may magnify the importance of that error, believing that he is a terrible AA member (reaffirming shame). Catastrophizing is popular among those with anxiety disorders who possess a propensity for combining cognitive distortions. Add some Fortune Telling to your Catastrophizing, and voila! What better way to increase stress than to imagine an awful outcome?

8. MINIMIZING

Minimization is incredibly common among those in active addiction or in early recovery. In speaking with someone pondering recovery from addiction, when asked about their consumption, patients will often use the words, *only*, *sometimes*, *a little* or other words intended to suggest that their problem is not as significant as it truly is — whether relating to frequency and amount of consumption or the consequences thereof. A person in recovery who receives their six-month medallion may minimize the importance of the milestone and continue believing that she is just lucky, thus denying herself a well-earned sense of accomplishment.

Self-awareness of this tendency enables us to own our problems so that we may put them into proper perspective, decreasing stress and increasing our resolve to address them.

9. EMOTIONAL REASONING

This may be one of the most important distortions to identify and address. Virtually all of us have bought into this distortion at one time or another. Emotional reasoning accepts one's emotions as facts. *I feel it, therefore it must be true.* Just because we feel something does not mean it is true; for example, we may become jealous and think our partner has feelings for someone else, but that does not make it true.

The intensity of emotions is a factor in emotional reasoning. The greater the emotion, the less the logic, resulting in consistently poor decisions. Those who struggle with codependency, relationship, or sex addictions may *feel* a strong connection with someone whom they have just met — and may treat that emotion of love, lust, or intrigue as a mutual fact to the exclusion of *actual* facts, leading to potential trouble. It is notable that boredom and loneliness (also emotions) are primary to most relapses. Emotional reasoning must be dealt with in real time if we are to consistently make good decisions with self-awareness and sound strategy.

10. IMPERATIVES

This damaging distortion is characterized by *should* statements made regarding ourselves or environmental factors. The clinical term is *imperatives,* which implies Rules. Rules about the way others, or we, or the world *should* be. I like to joke that people with a lot of imperatives *should* all over themselves and everyone around them. They impose a set of expectations that will likely not be met, and the result is often guilt or shame when we cannot live up to them.

When we are unaware of how imperatives impact our state of being, we are victimized twice over — once by our environment, and once by our lack of awareness. When we cling to *should* statements about ourselves, and others, they become a threat to our recovery. Irrational, self-directed imperatives make us feel badly about ourselves, undermining our self-esteem.

Dysfunctional family of origin and societal influences conspire to impose imperatives. Perfectionist parents with abundant *shoulds* are a source of anxiety, shame, and resentment for their children, from which alcohol and drugs provide relief.

Shoulds about our addictions can keep us from getting help out of stigma at identifying as one of *those people*.

Most have not undergone a full inventory of their own "shoulds". When we do, we will invariably find many that, upon closer examination, we will say to ourselves, "That's ridiculous! I don't believe that!"

Here's a simple example you may be able to relate to:

I am driving to my office and someone cuts me off. I experience anger and indignation. Nothing surprising there, right? But let us ponder the *shoulds* I *must* have in place behind that reflexive emotional cocktail. Note that some are rational, and others are not.

- After 60 years of practice, one *should* be better at driving.
- "Doesn't this lady know who I think I *am*?! She *should*!"
- The DMV personnel who administer driver licenses *should* always do their jobs perfectly, being such savvy, motivated personnel.
- Others *should* be able to read my mind (therefore knowing I have the right-of-way, regardless of circumstances).
- People *should* have eyes in the back of their heads.

- People of all ages *should* have a 100 percent flexible range of motion in order to be allowed to drive.
- My employer *should* fly me to work in a helicopter so I don't have to deal with these people.

I am sure there are more, but for our purposes this is sufficient to make the point . . .

If we are honest and thorough, we realize fairly quickly that a sense of humor is required to examine the beliefs underlying our emotions. Do I *really* believe all of those *shoulds* to be true? It must be so to explain the intensity of my indignant emotions.

One of the best short books I have read on maintaining our emotional center through identifying and resolving imperatives is, *12 Smart Things to Do When the Booze and Drugs Are Gone* by Alan Berger.

11. LABELING

These tendencies are basically an extreme form of overgeneralization, in which we assign judgments of value to ourselves or to others based on only one instance or experience, and apply a label. A student who labels herself as an idiot for failing an assignment, or a waiter who labels a customer a grumpy old fart for failing to thank the waiter for bringing his food is victim to this thinking error. Mislabeling applies highly emotional, loaded, and inaccurate or unreasonable language, with a lack of data points to support it. The main problem with this is that we are likely to miss out on positive experiences that those we have mislabeled may afford us.

An addict who relapses and then labels themselves a failure may promote a prolonged, covert relapse that could have ended sooner in the absence of self-labeling, and the stigma attached to it. In these cases, labeling reaffirms the addict's shame, impairing their resolve to use tools such as reaching out to others in recovery (the 100 lb. phone), attending 12-Step meetings, etc.

12. PERSONALIZING

Those who suffer from personalization are easily offended. As the name implies, this distortion involves taking everything personally.

The flip side of this coin would be assigning blame to yourself without any logical reason to believe you are to blame. In this sense, personalization covers a wide range of situations, from assuming you are the reason a friend did not enjoy the night out, to the more severe examples of believing that you are the cause for every instance of moodiness or irritation in those around you.

This distortion is usually expressed by disproportionately strong emotional responses to perceived slights, magnifying distress. Those with low self-esteem, such as those in early recovery, tend to own a lot of negative illusions. To them, *any* criticism feels like an existential threat. Perceived slights with no basis in reality occur throughout the day as the world goes about world-ing. In the absence of adequate data points, the individual with low self-esteem assumes the worst (Jumping to Conclusions), and then takes their unsubstantiated assumptions personally. Personalization is detrimental to the perpetrator as well as to those around them, needlessly undermining many relationships.

My mantra to those who take things personally is:

**Never confuse "me doing something for me"
as "me doing something to you."**

13. CONTROL FALLACY

Control Fallacy manifests as one of two beliefs: (1) that we either have *no* control over our lives and are helpless victims of our circumstances, or (2) that we are in *complete* control of ourselves and our surroundings and are thus responsible for all events and the feelings of those around us. Both beliefs are equally inaccurate.

Viktor Frankl's book entitled *Man's Search for Meaning* identifies attitudes useful to apply in situations where we feel victimized. Frankl was a Polish psychologist imprisoned in a concentration camp during WWII. His wife was killed in another camp, which only made things more difficult for him. His circumstances certainly qualified him to opine on how to navigate circumstances where we feel victimized. I often refer to his quotes in a clinical setting when patients feel victimized or painted into a corner:

> *When we are no longer able to change a situation, we are challenged to change ourselves.*

> *Everything can be taken from a man but one thing: the last of the human freedoms — to choose one's attitude in any given set of circumstances, to choose one's own way.*

> *It is not freedom from conditions, but it is freedom to take a stand toward the conditions.*

Control Fallacy is insidious in its capacity to perpetuate addiction. This is because if we believe that we are not in control of our emotional state, then it stands to reason that we are not responsible for our behaviors, particularly if the emotion is strong, such as lust, anger, or resentment. People tend to justify their reflexive responses citing *triggers,* therefore excusing themselves from accountability for engaging in their addictive behaviors. A classic version of this is, *You'd drink, too, if you were married to them!*

A more common word for Control Fallacy is *Blaming*.

Control Fallacy fails to acknowledge the period between emotion and action, thus the fault in logic.

Frankl states:

> *Between stimulus and response, there is a space. In that space is our power to choose our response. In our response lies our growth and our freedom.*

If we believe that others are responsible for our state of being, then we must also believe that we are responsible for others' emotional states, choices, and behaviors. After all, we are an environmental factor to them.

There is no shortage of people, usually codependents, who are happy to perpetuate this myth — those who believe, with good reason, that they can manipulate or *guilt* us into feeling responsible for their choices, thereby alleviating them of responsibility for their words and actions. Their assertion that we are responsible for their state and decisions justifies all kinds of self-righteous or abusive behavior.

We must realize that we are not victims unless we choose to be, in which case we are *still* not victims, because *victimhood, by definition, is a lack of choice.* When we understand this, and yet choose to portray ourselves as victims, we are being dishonest — to manipulate others.

Free Stuff!

I took *Algebra 1* three times during undergrad because I had to, passing only the last semester of my senior year with a D minus — minus. The professor felt sorry for me and passed me from the third attempt lest I return for another semester of college. That said, even I know that in any closed system there is only 100 percent to go around.

Behold *The First Law of Accountability* and its two corollaries — the remedy to Control Fallacy:

First, we need to understand and accept the *fact* that:

1. WE ARE *ALWAYS* 100 *PERCENT* RESPONSIBLE FOR OUR EMOTIONAL STATE OR CHOICES OR BEHAVIOR.

There is *only* 100 percent to go around, so it must then be true that:

1A) EVERYONE ELSE IS *ALWAYS* 0 *PERCENT* RESPONSIBLE FOR OUR EMOTIONAL STATE OR CHOICES OR BEHAVIOR.

And finally (the good news?):

1b) WE ARE *ALWAYS* 0 *PERCENT* RESPONSIBLE FOR OTHERS' EMOTIONAL STATE OR CHOICES OR BEHAVIOR.

I always tell my patients that if they simply internalized and lived this axiom, our work would be finished, and they could save thousands of dollars and a boatload of strife. Consider it a gift right now, from me to you. You're welcome.

14. FAIRNESS FALLACY

While we would all probably prefer to operate in a world that is fair, the assumption of a fair world is not based in reality. A person who judges every experience by perceived fairness is setting themselves up for unnecessary anger, resentment, and hopelessness when they inevitably encounter situations that are not fair.

The reason fairness is considered a fallacy is that there is no universal standard for fairness. Reasonable people can hold different standards for what is or is not fair — *insert any world conflict here.*

If parties can *agree* on what is and is not fair, that's a different story. Football games have rules and referees, but life for better or for worse is a minefield of differing rules and expectations, so a strong commitment to our own ideals for fairness sets us up for frustration and indignation that can serve to fuel relapse in the absence of adequate tools.

15. CHANGE FALLACY

This distortion is grounded in the belief that our happiness is contingent upon what other people either do, or don't do, or their circumstances.

If only _____ would do things in such-and-such a manner, or be a certain way, then I would be happy. The most overt sign of this fallacy is, for lack of a better word, *nagging.*

Every committed addict has experienced change fallacy from people trying to coerce them into changing into a person they find acceptable. And addicts, of course, rebut that they wouldn't drink so much were it not for the other's nagging.

Change fallacy feeds into itself, perpetuating frustration between any parties with no awareness of this cycle.

Attempting to change others — (1) breeds resentment, (2) gives others the idea that they are not worthy nor acceptable as they are, (3) does not work, (4) undermines relationships, and (5) causes unnecessary frustration.

There is a certain arrogance or self-centeredness in the idea that the world must conform to one's ideals, which is itself problematic.

My contention is that if you gave a person with Change Fallacy a magic wand with which they could make the world EXACTLY as they wanted it, within a matter of 5-10 minutes they would find something they wanted to change. These people are a moving target, possibly incapable of happiness under *any* circumstances.

The takeaway here is that happiness is always an inside job.

16. ALWAYS BEING RIGHT

Perfectionists and those with whom they associate recognize this distortion. It is the belief that we must always be right. Those struggling with this find the idea that they could be wrong unacceptable and will fight to the metaphorical death to prove they are right. A relatable example is internet commenters who spend hours arguing over an opinion or political issue beyond the point where reasonable individuals would decide to "agree to disagree".

This distortion is *usually* modeled by an adult or adults in the family-of-origin setting and can be devastating to the self-esteem of others in the family, particularly children.

The key to resolving this fallacy is to consult one's values and priorities, ultimately deciding whether the relationship is more important than *being right*.

17. HEAVEN'S REWARD FALLACY

This distortion plays out on big and small screens across the world daily. It is the false belief that one's struggles, suffering, and hard work will ultimately result in a just reward. Sadly, there are plenty of counterexamples available where hard work and sacrifice did not pay off.

Sometimes no matter how hard we work or sacrifice we will not achieve what we had hoped. For those with Heaven's Reward fallacy, this results in disappointment, frustration, anger, and even depression if the awaited reward does not materialize, creating fuel for potential relapse.

HOW THINKING ERRORS DESTROY RELATIONSHIPS IN EARLY RECOVERY

Cognitive distortions can be piggybacked on top of each other with compound results, and can jeopardize recovery, particularly in couples. The addicted aren't the only ones whose thought processes require examination. Many who have been in close relationships with someone during their active phase of addiction often develop thought processes involving multiple thinking errors, which, if not resolved, will not only cause them unnecessary distress, but will also destroy whatever remnants of their primary relationship remain. To illustrate one of the most common scenarios, I introduce to you Bitter Betty.

Bitter Betty likes to engage in what I refer to as the *triple-play*: 1) She engages in Mind Reading in the absence of data points, 2) takes what she conjures up Personally, and then 3) adds a little Emotional Reasoning to justify whatever comes out of her mouth. It is not difficult to envision the damage thinking errors impose on relationships — particularly addiction-plagued relationships in early recovery where emotional self-regulation is paramount for all involved.

Many codependents like Bitter Betty make inaccurate assumptions based on past experiences with their newly-recovering addicts, applying *formerly* valid assumptions to their loved one's new, unfamiliar behaviors. Attempting to impose control — the only coping mechanism they know — works to the mutual detriment of both parties because it undermines trust.

Early recovery is a tenuous state of abstinence. A codependent person not growing along with their loved one because of misplaced residual resentment, or a false belief that they needn't change (that it is not *their* problem), risks undermining the relationship.

Often as the addict in recovery becomes more self-sufficient, the codependent may begin to question their necessity to the recovering partner resulting in an irrational fear of abandonment. Without guidance, this experience can lead to back-sliding of the relationship into old dynamics, which increases the risk of relapse. Many couples who are pondering fundamental change, take comfort in their old ways because they, in the words of Joyce Myers, "... *may not like what's going on, but at least they know what's going on!*" The unfamiliar ground of new behaviors is disconcerting; so mutual participation is always the best policy in recovery for couples because they can navigate the change together.

A primary responsibility of a newly recovering person is to do whatever they must, in as authentic a manner as possible, to ensure their happiness while remaining mindful of the couple's mutual values. It is incumbent upon the codependent person to *not* take the recovering person's new, unfamiliar behaviors personally; but, instead learn to detach from the person who they *used* to fixate upon, finding their *own* happiness — regardless of what the recovering person is or is not doing.

If 95 percent of our stress is self-inflicted due to manifestation of the 17 common cognitive distortions, then that is the good news. Because anything self-inflicted can be self-remedied. With self-awareness and its strategic application, we are no longer dependent upon people nor circumstances to maintain our emotional center — our primary task in recovery.

We may now begin to practice catching ourselves *in real time* as our environment goes about doing what environments do — dishing out random circumstances. With practice, we transform from being victims to non-victims. When we had no understanding of detrimental unconscious programming, we were proverbial emotional leaves in the stream of life, reflexively bouncing off of life's events, people, and circumstances over which we have no control. Before gaining these insights, we were not running a program of any sort — our programming was running us — making us victims.

With time and practice, we are able to leverage these insights to the mutual benefit of ourselves, and those around us. We cease being our own worst enemy. Our thinking no longer works against us, and as such, we no longer feel as though we are constantly swimming upstream in our interactions with others — and with the world in general. Life is hard enough without self-inflicted thinking errors causing unnecessary strife.

In therapy, my patients work through all of the unforced errors contained in their Beliefs and Rules box. We identify and root out all of the imperatives that were unconsciously causing them anxiety and resentment that served as fuel for their addictions. We restore their true identity as individuals worthy of happiness and respect. We focus on future possibilities rather than remain fixated on past, limiting beliefs. We employ cognitive restructuring, applying traditional tools such as re-framing, exploring alternate explanations for upsetting circumstances, and increase self-awareness of their tendencies to default to worst-case scenarios when pondering their prospects. Old habitual thought processes die slowly; but, as patients expand their emotional intelligence with practice, they gain the ability to emotionally self-regulate. Navigating life and relationships becomes more intuitive; and, eventually these new mindsets become habitual, just as did the old, self-defeating ones.

Life becomes good again.

HOW "COGNITIVE RESTRUCTURING" WORKS

1	2	3	4
CIRCUMSTANCES	BELIEFS & RULES	EMOTIONS	CHOICES & BEHAVIORS
"Nouns" Environment People Events	THERAPY Re-Evaluate "Shoulds" Unhealthy Dependencies Unreasonable Expect. Re-Evaluate Self-Identity UNLIMITED POSSIBILITIES Correct Thinking Errors Re-Frame Circ. Alternate Explanations "Reality Check" Add A Time Element Worst-Case Scenarios Counter-Experiences Spirituality Purpose CONSULT OUR VISION Growth CONSULT VALUES	Decreased Intensity Curiosity HOPE Gratitude Relief Love Connection Confidence Pride Self-Esteem Intelligence Integrity Determination Vision	WAIT Don't Use Text a Friend Hit A Meeting Talk To Someone Loud Music Blissful Activity Get A Hug Meditate Call Parent Exercise Recreation Work Recovery Material Eat Something Swim

Our circumstances *plus* the meaning we assign our circumstances, yield an emotion which collectively informs our choices, which of course inform our circumstances, and the cycle continues indefinitely.

$$\vert: \big[(C + BR) \rightarrow E\big] \rightarrow CB :\vert$$

SUMMARY

STAGE 1 RECOVERY — PREVENT RELAPSE

+ Cognitive distortions are the underlying logic to which we attach our beliefs, and the facts of our circumstances, to make meaning of them. Faulty logic, which causes about 95 percent of our distress, is an *unforced error*. Resolving this, decreases stress, and thus, relapse potential.

+ Identifying and resolving our most egregious *thinking errors* enables us to:

> Regulate our emotions, resulting in better decisions.
>
> Take full responsibility for our actions.
>
> Increase confidence and self-esteem as we become able to guarantee our behavior.

+ To catch ourselves falling into these *thinking errors* in real time is exhilarating. Emotional self-regulation becomes a passion as we gain success avoiding the pitfalls to which we previously fell victim.

STAGE 2 RECOVERY — REGAIN AUTHENTICITY

+ As we gain experience in managing our emotional state, we start reaping benefits such as healthy relationships. We become willing to take greater risks in authenticity, and are more comfortable in our own shoes. With success comes the desire to further assert our authenticity, creating an upward trend.

+ Asserting authenticity disconfirms preconceptions we may have had about how others perceive us. These experiences self-perpetuate the desire to take greater and greater risks at showing our True Self.

STAGE 3 RECOVERY — ENHANCE SPIRITUAL CAPACITY

+ As we become more resilient, we become less shame-based, and feel less victimized by our circumstances. The increased sense of self and power makes the concept of adopting a spiritual perspective easier to swallow.

+ Deciding to engage a spiritual dimension out of choice feels much better than doing so out of desperation. We know that we can still trust ourselves if things don't work out, making the risk of trusting a higher power less daunting.

HOW AUTHENTICITY WORKS

WILL THE REAL [YOUR NAME HERE] PLEASE STAND UP?

If you have not yet reviewed this video lecture by Dr. Gabor Mate' (3.1 in Chapter 3), please do so now. The points applied in Chapter 3 relate to the connection between the brain and physiology, particularly how these factors conspire to impact emotions, and conversely, how our emotions impact our physiology in the long term. But this mind and body connection is also critical in restoring authenticity, which, in turn, is critical in restoring self-esteem, and our ability to connect with any higher power.

 6.1

Our identity consists of unquestioned beliefs we hold about who we are, and are not. In childhood our identity was determined by how we perceived that our parent(s) perceived us. As young children, we did not have the capacity to critically analyze the accuracy of our parents' assessment of us. All we knew was that, from an evolutionary perspective, being unacceptable to a parent was not an option. After all, our 3-year-old-logic told us, if we were unacceptable to our parents we would not be loved. And if we were not loved we would be abandoned. And if we were abandoned we would die. So, early on we learned to repress aspects of our personality that our parents signaled were unacceptable. This adaptation for survival was necessary because the human infant is by far the most dependent of any creature on the planet (and for the longest period of time). So, without attachment, there is no life.

Most children grow out of their fear-based need to remain attached at any cost. But a vast majority of the population with whom I work have found that this fear-based relational dynamic never left them. This codependency informed all of their relationships from childhood throughout adulthood. Clinically speaking, this fear-based pathology yields low self-esteem over time through continuous denial of their True Self.

Gabor Mate' states that all emotional pathology is rooted in whether or not as a child our emotional needs were met. He points out that if as children we were neglected, abused, invalidated, discounted, or not honored by our parents through overt, or discreet messaging, the result is always shame and a people-pleasing personality, which, left unchecked, confers a life sentence of shame-based misery.

The following constitute significant risk factors for addiction, anger issues, codependence, depression, and chronic, immune-related illnesses in an individual:

- Automatic and compulsive regard for the emotional needs of others while ignoring his or her own.
- Automatic and rigid identification with Duty, Role, and Responsibility over the needs of the self.
- Repression of so-called negative emotions, particularly anger.
- Belief that he or she is responsible for how other people feel.
- Belief that he or she should never disappoint anyone — that they should never say "no."

Over 80 percent of my patients, at any given point in time, identify with most of these risk factors to the extent that they rank the strength of their identification with them on average between 7-10 on a scale of 1-10 (10 being highest). The by-product of strong identification with these attributes is *always* resentment.

RESENTMENT

Spend enough time in the rooms of AA, and we learn that resentment is rocket fuel for addiction and relapse. As such, there is no place for resentment in the life of a person in recovery. Resentment justifies all kinds of egregious behavior — I know — and lived this all too well.

But why the resentment? The risk factors listed above appear at face value to be positive, compassionate attitudes.

The answer is that there is a survival instinct equally as strong as the need for attachment — Authenticity. Authenticity is directly connected to gut instincts — knowing who we are, and what we want. A human infant knows exactly what it wants, and is willing to do whatever is necessary to acquire its needs because it is completely in touch with its gut instincts. Gut instincts enable us to determine who and what is *safe* — a survival mechanism that precedes our ability as a species to even think.

Dr. Gabor Mate' asks, "What if the need for Authenticity threatens the need for attachment (to the parent)?" On one hand, the child wants what it wants; but, if a parent is a rage-aholic, or has disproportionately angry responses to the child's authentic needs, the child represses their Authenticity as an adaptation to survive. Mate' asserts the repression of Authenticity in favor of attachment — and associated cumulative resentment — is the root cause of all emotional pathology moving forward, including addiction.

Repression of the True Self has another name — dishonesty.

Dishonesty comes in two classes — active and passive — both of which eat away at our self-esteem like termites on a wood foundation. Active dishonesty is the garden variety type — lie, cheat, or steal. Passive dishonesty is more insidious, although both deplete self-esteem.

Passive dishonesty occurs every time we smile when we feel like crying; every time we say *yes* when we really mean *no*; every time we work when we really need or want to play. Whenever we acquiesce to *keep the peace*, passive dishonesty occurs and Authenticity is repressed. Over years or even decades, the cumulative resentment amassed becomes a cesspool of anger fueling addictive behaviors and undermining self-esteem.

Our Inner Child is approximately the same age we were when we began self-repressing for the purpose of maintaining attachment with our parents. In most people, that is about 3 years of age.

When describing the Inner Child to group members in guided meditations, I have them imagine a filthy little 3-year-old child huddled in a dark, torch-lit, dirt-floored dungeon with an old-school chalkboard on wheels in the middle of the room. They visualize this grubby, neglected Inner Child standing there with dirt on his or her face and a stub of chalk in his or her hand. Every time we say "yes" when we mean "no," or acquiesce out of fear of abandonment, the child puts a tally mark on the chalkboard. And the chalkboard is already completely full of tally marks accumulated over decades of denying the self, in order to maintain attachment to those we were fearful of losing. As a result, the child hates us — and who could blame it when we have denied its existence and importance as our True Self?! By this 3-year-old Inner Child's logic, if we were not ashamed of him or her, why would we deny its existence, keeping it tucked away in a filthy dungeon where no one can see it?!

When we habitually marginalize our Inner Child — our True Self — in favor of attachment, the messages we are giving it (and thus, ourselves) are: *You don't count. You're not worthy of consideration. No one cares, or should care what you think. You're not important. You don't matter. You're embarrassing. No one wants you.*

Later relationships with spouses, significant others, etc., whose marginalizing ways felt *familiar* to us reaffirmed the shaming messages we were gifted with as young children. In *their* absence, we have our very own Inner Critic taking up the slack in perpetuating our shame.

Those with people-pleasing personalities tend to attract abusive, manipulative, controlling, narcissistic, or self-centered partners who are more than happy to take advantage of the people-pleaser's fear of abandonment. A person with low self-esteem is, to a narcissist's delight, eminently controllable through threat of abandonment, either directly or indirectly, or through degrading verbal abuse. The abuser knows the people-pleaser will absorb the abuse because it matches their Identity. Remember, the abuser is simply telling the individual with low self-esteem something that reaffirms that which they already believe to be true about themselves.

When a people-pleasing person realizes their fear-based pathology has kept them in abusive relationships — or more likely in a string of them throughout their lifetime — their reaction usually includes anger at themselves, and fierce resolve to regain their autonomy, dignity, and self-esteem. As a therapist there is little more satisfying than being a catalyst and witness to such healthy change in patients. The narcissistic partner often finds this new-found autonomy unwelcome. The outcome of the relationship is largely predicated upon the formerly controlling party's willingness to undergo their own healthy changes. I would speculate on the probability of this occurring, but it's impossible to do so, having been surprised on many occasions at outcomes differing from my predictions.

There ought to be small print at the bottom of therapeutic intake forms that says, *If you succeed in making the changes you say you want to make going into this therapeutic episode, there may be unintended consequences.*

I recently had a patient referred by their significant other who did not like how the patient's drinking affected relational dynamics between them. As I got to know the patient and her patterns, it became clear that the significant other who referred the patient to me actually preferred the patient's substance use over her new-found abstinence-based autonomy. The patient could be more easily controlled through shame, guilt, and threats of abandonment when drinking. The referrer became disillusioned with the process, and for a period, convinced the patient to discontinue therapy. However, a seed had been planted, leaving the referrer the choice to become the kind of person the patient would *want* to be around, or face losing the relationship.

In the end, the referrer was unable to adjust, resenting the idea that *he* should have to change when it was the *patient* who had the problem, in his eyes. The ending to this story has yet to be written. As a therapist, it is not my job to advocate for a particular outcome relationally. It is to help my client navigate whatever outcome he or she selects with coping tools to succeed at accomplishing their outcome while maintaining recovery.

HOW INAUTHENTICITY DOES NOT WORK

Regaining one's authenticity is a major theme in recovery. What we are recovering in Recovery is our authenticity — our True Self, which was abandoned, forgotten, and neglected early in life — but who is still in there waiting for us to recognize him or her.

Many self-proclaimed people-pleasers suffer from what Alan Berger, in his book, *12 Smart Things to Do When the Booze and Drugs Are Gone* does a great job illustrating: Bonsai Tree Syndrome. Berger describes one of the core issues behind low self-esteem and thus addiction: Passive Dishonesty, which results in a discrepancy between our True Self and the False Self we believe necessary to be lovable to others.

> *Have you ever seen a beautiful bonsai tree? A bonsai artist works patiently over many years to constrain what should be a full-sized tree into perfect miniature. The artist constantly prunes the tree, wraps wires around its branches to shape them, deprives it of water, and trims its roots to fit a tiny pot.*
>
> *Such a tree becomes perfect to look at. And yet . . . and yet. It is not its true-self. It is a tree made to conform to a vision of miniature perfection.*
>
> *Every one of us was anxious or hurt in some form as a child — whether real or perceived, and we developed an image of how we*

should be in order for the world to love us — a set of rules that, if followed, would make us "perfect."

If we are honest, we will see that our rules have made bonsai of us — bonsai of the soul. We are so afraid that our true-self is unlovable that we coil our soul with wire, drink just enough water to stay alive — but never enough to quench — and trim our roots. Like the bonsai artist, we spend years warping our true-self into a false-self. A few of us are masters at this, and we seem, to others, to be perfect.

But the reality is that we have constrained our true-self in an attempt to be loved. This is the impact of our perfectionist spec-ifications — to warp our true selves to fit the rules we think will make us lovable.

The bonsai'd soul is the false-self. No human can live in such self-made bondage without breaking out now and then. And when we do, we act out in frightening ways — often in ways that betray the perfect false-self we have worked so hard to create.

In emotional recovery, we learn to remove the coils, to drink enough water, and to plant our souls in earth that is rich and large enough to nurture us and mature us. And we learn to accept that some of our branches will be beautiful, and some will be scarred, and some will be laughable. We learn that as we learn to accept our true-self.

Many incorrectly believe that self-esteem is some sort of ambig-uous, mercurial concept requiring an equally oblique solution. This is simply false. The best and fastest way to restore self-esteem is *honesty*. Not just by not lying, but by actively asserting our True Self. Honesty takes courage and practice, but is *the* antidote to low self-esteem. The aforementioned risk factors Gabor Mate' identifies for chronic illness, and which I identify as precursors to resentment and thus addiction, are all loving, compassionate attitudes.

- Automatic and compulsive regard for the emotional needs of others while ignoring his or her own.
- Automatic and rigid identification with Duty, Role, and Responsibility over the needs of the self.
- Repression of so-called negative emotions, particularly anger.
- Belief that he or she is responsible for how other people feel.
- Belief that he or she should never disappoint anyone — that they should never say "no."

But without healthy boundaries, they mark the undoing of our self-esteem. Patients who rank the degree to which they identify with them at an 8-10 on a scale of 1-10 (10 being highest) need to dial these noble impulses back to a healthy 4-5 level.

We must value and honor ourselves even though this feels unfamiliar; and, as we begin to reap the benefits of asserting our authenticity, we will *never* want to go back to our old ways.

Mutual support groups such as ACA afford us the gift of a safe environment in which to practice being rigorously vulnerable without judgment. In short order, we begin to generalize this experience outside the therapeutic environment. Our confidence surges as we learn that we can assert ourselves without shame.

Many, whether in active addiction, in recovery, and even those with no substance-related issues, have no idea what Authenticity *feels* like. They have often forgotten who they are. One of the sadder conversations I have with patients (and have had with myself) is when they realize that they have *never* experienced a truly loving, healthy relationship. Often, the closest thing those afflicted with addictions have experienced relationally is a codependent, enmeshed, fear-based relationship. When you're 30, 40, 50, etc. years old, learning this can be painful.

Those afflicted with significant shame present a strong False Self. This is a defense mechanism designed to keep others from seeing their True Self, which sadly also keeps them from experiencing true love. The False Self is perfected throughout the patient's life to the extent that they can be surrounded by friends who adore them, and yet be lonely. Consider the rock stars and comedians who have killed themselves via drugs or alcohol at the pinnacle of their career. They were unable to be authentic, so any validation they received never hit home. They painted a picture (a False Self) to deflect from the True Self they intuitively believed did not deserve love. Tragic.

REGAINING AUTHENTICITY

Vulnerability is the antidote to shame. Dr. Brené Brown does an excellent job of describing what authenticity (vulnerability) looks like in a Ted Talk (6.2). I use her definition of Love: "Human connection as a result of authenticity." Love need not come from one source — although this belief is a common misconception among the codependent. We can receive love from many sources. In fact, the therapeutic environment is the embodiment of love in the sense that it involves two people relating (hopefully) their true selves. I tell patients that ideally they will recreate a therapeutic-like setting with friends and loved ones outside of the office environment. The extent to which they accomplish this is the degree to which they will experience love from multiple sources (as opposed to *putting all of their (emotional) eggs in one basket,* such as in a primary relationship).

Brené Brown's Ted Talk (6.2) explains how vulnerability is the antidote to shame, and how it clears the way to accessing our

True Self. She explains that the opposite of a shame-based person is a *wholehearted* person — a completely foreign concept to those afflicted with addiction or in early recovery.

 6.2

Asserting our authenticity is an *experiential* intervention. It is only through the *act* of being vulnerable and stating true things about ourselves — many self-perceived as shameful — and surviving the experience, that we gain confidence. ACA meetings provide the best format for this experience.

One of the overriding meeting rules is *no crosstalk,* which means no one may comment on, add to, nor reference anyone else's share during the meeting. This dynamic creates a perfect environment in which to practice vulnerability. Many tears are shed in these meetings, often accompanied by words to the effect that, "I don't know why I'm crying." The crying represents tears of relief from the Inner Child who is *finally* being heard after often decades of repression by the False Self.

Dr. Brown relates that a *wholehearted* person intuitively feels as though they deserve love while the *ashamed* do not. Nor do those in addiction or in early recovery. The *ashamed* only accept messages that match our true, shame-based self-image. As such, the only way to begin receiving love is to change our identity — the unquestioned set of beliefs we have about ourselves that cause us to deny love and validation while embracing self-deprecating messages.

We are all inherently lovable and worthy of love. We need to learn by experience to believe it. Therapy, participation in ACA meetings, and in other mutual support groups, provides multiple opportunities to assert authenticity in a safe environment.

It's worth reiterating that only in a state of *being* our True Self are we able to restore self-esteem, and commune with a higher power beyond a saccharine, intellectualizing level. Having the courage to assert our authenticity is something new to us. But we signed up for change, right? If we truly want what we *say* we do, then we are going to have to do things differently than we used to.

Many are afraid of losing relationships when we become more authentic, and we very well may. As we begin to practice asserting our authenticity, some people are undoubtedly going to rotate out of our lives, and those losses may hurt temporarily. However, other people who see our True Selves will love and accept us, replacing those who provided validation of our False Self, which was unsatisfying anyway.

When we muster the courage to show who we are, others' validation hits home, because they can actually see the target. As time progresses, and we gain experience living in Authenticity, not only does our self-esteem grow, but an unfamiliar confidence surfaces.

We assert authenticity in a manner similar to that in which a bat uses echolocation to navigate its environment. Feedback received serves as data that helps us discern who is *safe*, and who is not, so that we may navigate our social environment. As our self-esteem improves, feedback feels more like data than judgment, as it does for anyone not afflicted with a shame-based identity. Our skin is no longer so thin. Things that seem like rejection no longer feel like an existential threat.

As we gain true friends, we realize that we need not possess everyone we love, because we are no longer afraid they will abandon us. Ability to derive love from any relationship is a protective factor, because in doing so, it is impossible for any single person to devastate us by threatening to withhold validation or approval. This inoculates us against narcissists who would want to control us or bend us into a bonsai tree.

BECOMING A SAFE PERSON TO LOVE

As we define and assert our boundaries, we become safer to love.

Transitioning from the False Self, which we thought we had to be in order to be lovable to others, to our authentic True Self, which I refer to as the *Authentication Process*, is likely to be painful, at least temporarily. Thankfully this is a one-time experience, most of which may be accomplished in a relatively short time frame — perhaps months — with proper effort, guidance, and courage.

Undoubtedly, those with whom we have surrounded ourselves over the years have become used to our reflexive accommodation to *their* agenda, and will throw fits as we become more autonomous and confident in asserting our True Self. It is difficult to hold them in contempt for asserting their controlling instincts because, after all, we trained them to expect us to be extensions of them. Stakeholders in the status quo will call us selfish, condescending, and uncaring as they attempt to shame us back into submission. Our reflexive response is often guilt at asserting our self-will. But we *must* leverage every available resource to keep on track throughout the Authentication Process. Such resources may include daily reflection readings, individual or group therapy, ACA meetings, guided meditation, and communion with fellow travelers on our journey. We must not waver.

In moving toward our ideal state of being, and asserting our True Self, people who knew us prior to beginning the Authentication Process are either going to adapt, or leave. Unfortunately, some unable to adapt will be spouses, family members, friends, and employers. The thought of this is terrifying.

Why is this? Well, we probably have little or no experience dealing with relationship losses while sober. The loss of my first primary relationship while sober nearly killed me — literally. My Cabin Story in Chapter 7 recounts this dark episode.

It is also likely that our default inclination is to assume that no one will love us for who we truly are, based on past experience. This belief is false. It is an illusion, and simply knowing this in advance is beneficial. Although our unlovability may have been our perception in childhood, perhaps justified, it is important to remember two things: 1) that was *then*, and this is *now*, and 2) we have probably never given anyone the opportunity to either love or reject our True Self since childhood. This is due to our perceived need to not present authentically to others out of fear of rejection, which, if risked, would reaffirm our childhood belief that we are unlovable.

Quitting drugs and alcohol was difficult, but necessary. Since April 26, 2014, my sobriety has been my single most prized possession. I will *not* sacrifice, nor exchange it for anyone's approval, even under threat of abandonment. Now, having engaged in the Authentication Process, my Authenticity has been added to the list of things I will *never* give up. If my sobriety is my most prized possession, becoming and asserting the best possible version of my True Self has become my primary focus.

Those in relationships with people in addiction know that they are involved with a moving target where uncertainty is more the rule than the exception. I have had many patients' counterparts refer to a Jeckyl and Hyde personality when describing their partner. This is due to the emotional unpredictability symptomatic of addiction. As my True Self, I am no longer a moving target. I know who I am, and as such I am not likely to change much, which makes me safer to love, both in the immediate, and in the future.

The ACA *Big Red Book* notes that living in an authentic state of being — the True Self — provides an ideal gateway to spirituality.

There is a certain poetry in the notion that our only way to spirituality is by way of our inner child, the gatekeeper who has been continually abused by everyone, including ourselves, for its entire life. Until we recover our authentic self, and heal our inner child, our ability to connect with our future Ideal Self is impaired.

Trust and vulnerability are hard to come by when we possess an inner child who was subjected to repression and marginalization for decades. Joseph Campbell's hero's journey, with which we will soon become aquainted, is completed by recovering our authenticity. This is the final, most difficult battle that *must* be won in order to gain the holy grail, which in our case, is the means to connect with a higher power. Foes to be defeated along this journey include dysfunctional family members; narcissistic partners whose ways felt familiar; addiction; shame; and our inner critic who always took up the cause following the defeat of these other antagonists.

For many in recovery, regaining and then asserting their authenticity is possibly the most scary thing they have ever done. The "what-if" questions are terrifying! *What if I am my True Self, and I am rejected? Could I survive that?* Those who overcome these obstacles are truly heroes.

Living in alignment with our true values, engaging in appropriate therapeutic interventions, and regular attendance of ACA meetings where the "no cross-talk" rules prevail, provide patients many benefits associated with restored authenticity, including:

- Increased Self-Esteem
- Decreased Anxiety
- Decreased Depression
- Confidence

- Clarity of Purpose
- Worthiness of Love
- Fearlessness
- Connection to Others
- Safe to Love

BECOMING YOUR TRUE SELF

This process of transitioning from addiction and spiritual skepticism involves peeling away layers of pathology — first addiction and other mental health issues, and then shame. In order to affect lasting recovery from addiction, our shame-based identity must change. UTR expedites this process.

It is a fact of nature that we are in a constant state of flux. Our cells are constantly dying and being replaced by new ones. The atoms that comprise the molecules that our cells are made up of consist of subatomic particles that appear, disappear, and then reappear nearly instantaneously as energy levels fluctuate. In reality, the only thing keeping us the same person we were three seconds ago is our memory of whom we are supposed to be, as defined by environmental factors we consult throughout our waking hours that *remind* us of our identity: emails, calendars, social media posts, other people, etc.

Dispenza often makes the point that, "In order to have a new personal reality, we need a new personality." Such a change in personality would undoubtedly yield a new personal reality — both internally in thought, and externally by virtue of how we would interact with our environment. We are unlikely to sustain change as the same personality from whence the status quo evolved. *We literally must become someone else.*

For those in recovery from addiction, that *someone else* must be our True Self, or Inner Child. That's good news because our True Self is already there inside of each of us. It never left — it's just been buried by years of neglect and dysfunction. But it's there; and, it contains the basis for our highest aspirations.

HOW IDENTITY WORKS

Many of us become skeptical of our future prospects as we ponder our failed efforts at change from the past. We incorrectly weigh past failures in calculating our future prospects. Yet, we have never attempted to change our reality from the perspective of being a different person. Nor have we taken quantum field theory into account — but let's not get ahead of ourselves.

We all have the same hardware — a presumably functional brain and sensory apparatus. We have our belief system or worldview — the human version of a computer's operating system. Had my software programming been more closely aligned with Sir Richard Branson's there is no question that many aspects of my life would be different than they are at the moment.

Our beliefs about *who we are*, are so deeply ingrained that even our physiology reinforces them. This is why it is difficult to establish and maintain fundamental change. When we go from being a person in active addiction to being a person in sustained recovery, those states of being are completely alien to each other. The person in active addiction is, in fact, a different person than one in recovery — as evidenced by how they unconsciously (and consciously) process environmental factors, such as people and events and their ensuing behavior.

Our overall goal is to become an idealized version of our True Self, completely realizing our full potential. Caroline McHugh makes an argument for becoming the best possible version of ourselves in the following TedTalk:

 6.3

This talk makes a number of fascinating distinctions, but one of the most useful is the importance of developing what she calls an *Interiority Complex* (yes, I spelled that correctly).

McHugh points out that many of us have an inferiority complex by which we compare ourselves with others whom we perceive as being superior. Not surprisingly, this results in a negative self-assessment, which undermines self-esteem. Others suffer from a superiority complex, an overactive ego, which serves to disconnect them from others who are perceived unworthy of connection. This undermines the interdependence necessary for sustained recovery. The common denominator with both superiority and inferiority complexes is that they are *other-centered*. They require others in order to apply value judgments about ourselves.

McHugh suggests that it is healthier to develop an *interiority complex*. In this state, she posits, we compare ourselves not to others or their standards, but to our past self and an envisioned future version of ourselves where our potential is fully realized. This is a way to measure our progress on the journey to becoming our best self, our True Self.

One of McHugh's most salient points is that the most outstanding people in the world and throughout history (of whom she has studied) all have *one* thing in common: *nothing*. This reinforces the importance of authenticity, not just for the individual, but for everyone on the planet.

Stage 1 Recovery Bonus: This perspective decreases anxiety because in adopting it, we are no longer competing with anyone

— only with our past self. We are 100 percent in control of this competition. There is intrinsic, and *extrinsic,* value in all of us becoming the best possible version of ourselves. One cannot help but ask the question, *What would the world be like if we all fearlessly pursued our best selves oblivious of the social pressures imposed by society and others?*

WHAT UTR DOES FOR US

With UTR we don't leave our destiny (nor the personality required to live it) to chance. We create it. So if we are going to go to the trouble of designing a new personality, why not consciously choose values and beliefs we believe will provide the most satisfying experiences imaginable? For this, we need look no further than our Inner Child — our True Self — in designing a personality and life where the predominant emotion from the time we wake up in the morning until the time we go to sleep is *gratitude*. This vision originates from our True Self — the mechanics of which are fascinating, and will be thoroughly discussed in Part II of this book.

During this design process we develop clarity about which attributes no longer serve us. Fears about what others might think, abandonment, rejection, judgment, or anything that causes us to discount our True Self are shed. When our outside and inside match, the opportunity exists to be loved and accepted for who we are.

We embody the belief that *it is far better to be rejected for who we are than to be loved for who we are not.*

For many, this is enough. Authenticity is one of the conditions necessary to engage in healthy relationships. When we change ourselves, everything around us changes. If we — or our True Self — can't be seen and experienced by others, how can we possibly say that we are having a relationship?

When we become our True Self, the right people will enter our lives, and love us for who we are. There is no substitute for this kind of connection, and it is the basis for True Love, whether human or spiritual.

SUMMARY

STAGE 1 RECOVERY — PREVENT RELAPSE

+ Experiencing and asserting authenticity aligned with our innate identity reduces stress.
+ There is a transitional period where others may reject our new True Self as we assert authenticity. This is one of the most challenging aspects of recovery, and can cause us to backslide due to the discomfort of unfamiliarity. Therefore, during these periods of growth, we must lean on those in recovery for support. Healthy interdependence boosts resilience against relapse.
+ Clearly defined boundaries make us safer to love.
+ True Love (as a result of authenticity) *always* increases resilience and decreases relapse potential.
+ If, in our authenticity, others leave us, it is not because we are defective or unlovable. Understanding this helps us maintain our emotional center, and be more resilient to what we used to interpret as rejection.

STAGE 2 RECOVERY — REGAIN AUTHENTICITY

+ Our False Self was an adaptation based upon the false belief that we had to be something other than our True Selves in order to be lovable. This belief was usually imposed during childhood.
+ Vulnerability is the greatest measure of courage, and is not a weakness.

+ The one thing *all* of the most outstanding people in the world have in common is *Nothing*.
+ As we gain experience in unapologetically asserting our authenticity, we become more aware of our past, fear-based dishonesty. The consequent disgust drives us toward self realization.

STAGE 3 RECOVERY — ENHANCE SPIRITUAL CAPACITY

+ As we assert ourselves authentically, we intuitively become aware of our intrinsic value, enabling us to feel worthy of the consideration of a higher power.
+ When we assert our True Selves, we begin to receive feedback from the Universe that we are headed in the right direction — bolstering our faith therein.
+ Feedback from the Universe reinforces our resolve to continue our journey and to ponder *what else is possible in an authentic state*.
+ In dealing with imperfect human beings, we will realize that a source of love and acceptance that does not abandon us is useful — the kind of love and acceptance given by a divine source — motivating us to continue to seek such a source.

CHAPTER 7

HOW MOTIVATION WORKS

One axiom in my field is that an addict is not going to change unless faced with the prospect of losing something they are not willing to live without. Loved ones are often floored to learn that *they* are not the something their loved one is unwilling to live without. As this becomes apparent, loved ones experience not only the possible loss of a valuable relationship, but also the loss of their dreams, as their hoped-for future disintegrates before them.

At such times, I have found it useful to quote Eckhart Tolle, pointing out that their ideas of the future are just that — mirages with no real basis in reality. Just as any dismal future they conjure up, based on their loved one's struggles with addiction, is not real.

> *People don't realize that now is all there ever is. There is no past nor future except as memory or anticipation in your mind.*

Stakeholders, and those afflicted with addiction, need to understand that, as with stock investments, *past performance does not guarantee future results.* This reality is essential for addicts and loved ones to internalize. We will explore the reasons for this in Part II.

Codependent people have it worse than the addicted person since they often do not use substances to numb their feelings; and so they have full emotional access to the pain, frustration, fear, and resentment that comes from being a person who loves someone in active addiction. My work with them involves learning how to detach with love, and how to best maintain *their* emotional center regardless of the addicted person's choices or behavior.

There is another principle in my line of work: *Never work harder than your patients*. We cannot get, or stay, sober for them. The same applies to stakeholders in an addict's life. While caretaking is often ingrained in a codependent's personality, this trait must be resolved. Codependents engage in multiple distortions: Control Fallacy, Change Fallacy, Fortune-Telling (Mind-Reading), Imperatives, and Catastrophization chief among them. Working with a therapist to eliminate these distortions is instrumental for a codependent person for there to be hope of reconciliation with a person in recovery. In cases where a codependent's relationship with an addict is beyond repair, in the absence of therapy they will enter into an identical relationship with someone possessing the same behaviors as their former addict — same person, different name, because it *feels* familiar. It is never a coincidence that addicts and codependent people find each other. Addicts need caretakers, and caretakers need projects. A codependent person *must* put themselves into a position where they will not repeat the same (unconscious) mistakes that led them into the misery they just left.

MOVING FROM EXTERNAL TO INTERNAL MOTIVATION

The longevity of fundamental change is contingent upon the locus of motivation. External motivation doesn't work for long.

Addicts must come to their *own* realization that the *discrepancy* between the life that they are experiencing and that of which they are capable is no longer acceptable. Usually, someone entering treatment is *externally* motivated by a stakeholder in their life — employer, partner, parent, etc. It is incumbent upon a therapist to help clients convert this locus of motivation to internal. Anyone externally motivated can change long enough to get someone off their back. But the by-product of external motivation, as we have learned, is always resentment, which invariably results in retaliation in the form of using or drinking *at* the person or circumstances for whom they are changing, as warranted by their twisted addicted logic.

Lasting change requires internal motivation.

Thankfully, most humans are aspirational in nature. They instinctively strive to grow. The tension between the current level of an addict's functionality, and that of which they know they are capable, must be harnessed if lasting change is to be expected.

The first step in UTR is to develop a future vision so compelling that *not* moving toward it is out of the question. This is the purpose of the *Magic Wand Thought Experiment* outlined later.

Internal motivation is guided by values and beliefs about our Identity. Those in active addiction can be internally motivated, but by corrupt, *addictive* values like dishonesty, self-centeredness, entitlement, and disregard for the emotional well-being of anyone else.

HOW RECOVERY STARTS

I was not externally motivated when admitted to The Betty Ford Center in 2014. Nor was I internally motivated by a desire to become the best possible version of myself. By the time I went to treatment, my innate values had been overwritten by years of addiction. The addiction-based values I had adopted after 18 years of heavy substance use were not consistent with my innate values. I was not motivated to regain my reputation with myself and others, nor did I care to become a safe person to love. In addiction, the corrupt values of the False Self that serve as a defense mechanism *underlying* addiction, grow and prevail.

Any internal motivation at that time was predicated upon the negative values I had honed throughout my chronic addiction — particularly greed — one of the internal values of the False Self that flourishes in the dark.

My thinking went something like this:

1. My parents are getting old.

2. I am faced with the prospect of losing a legacy-sized inheritance due to their judgmental (stigma) attitude associated with addiction — particularly in light of the sordid details of my life leading up to the wheels falling off.

3. I believe they're smart enough to understand that one of the best ways to kill someone in active addiction is to give them a few million bucks.

4. Therefore, I should go through treatment.

So, my plan as I entered treatment became:

A. Divorce my wife so I can,

B. move in with my hot stripper girlfriend whom I had been dating for eight months prior to admission to treatment,

C. wait my folks out — sober if necessary — until they die,

D. offer to provide random drug tests if necessary, to ensure their trust, and then

E. go back to my partying ways with tons of money, a hot girlfriend, and my life would be restored to its former glory, times ten.

Upon further reflection a more honest assessment of my motives would be that I was motivated by fear of being penniless or even more accurately, fear of abandonment due to being penniless. In other words, I wasn't nefarious, evil, and cunning — I was pathetic, afraid, and had unfathomably low self-esteem. The fact of the matter is that I overidentified with having money to the extent that my only value (in my mind at the time, at least) lay in whatever was in my wallet.

Not surprisingly, when the money ran out so did everyone else, at which point I reasoned it best to kill myself — ironically, with more drugs and alcohol.

The plan to get sober so I could show my folks it was alright to keep me in their will didn't last long. I awoke after spending one night at The Betty Ford Center thinking, *You know what, screw this, and everyone. I'll just take my chances.* At that point my *new* plan became to move in with my girlfriend and deal cocaine to make ends meet. True insanity, even in the absence of substances for 18 hours.

What took place next is actually a good story that also contains two critical milestones in my early recovery process:

> *I awoke after the first night in Ottenstein Hall, the medically supervised wing of The Betty Ford Center that houses those entering treatment to be treated for acute physical withdrawal.*
>
> *I looked at the goodie bag on the bedside table that they had given me at admission. It included an* Alcoholics Anonymous

Big Book *and an AA tome entitled, "The Twelve Steps and Twelve Traditions of Alcoholics Anonymous" aka the "Twelve by Twelve." I had seen these books before, as they were the very same ones I'd been given at age 17 when I went through my first stint in treatment. I thought to myself, 'This is bullshit,' and I began packing the duffel bag I'd hastily packed before being hauled off to treatment.*

I had no money, as I'd left with just my wallet, the contents of which I'd spent the day before on my last hurrah. I had apparently requested some money be transferred to my bank from my brokerage firm (that was going to take three days because I had to sell some stocks that had to settle first). The only thing of value I did have was my Omega watch that I'd gotten in the Bahamas — one of my prized possessions. But regardless, I figured I'd walk into town (Rancho Mirage), pawn the watch, which should net me a few thousand dollars, buy a train ticket back to Los Angeles, and move in with my girlfriend to start dealing. Easy peasy.

As I walked across the beautifully-manicured grounds toward the security gate, Jimmy Weiss — whose euphemistic job title was, "Patient Advocate" — came hustling, double-time, out of Firestone Hall, which was where his office was, and flagged me down. (Apparently, I'm not the only person in the history of The Betty Ford Center who decided the day after they got into treatment that maybe this wasn't for them.) So, Jimmy asked me to come to his office for a few minutes, and I figured, 'Why not, nothing to lose'.

Jimmy's office was interesting. One thing I noticed right away was an electric guitar he had on the wall, which gave him some credibility with me, as I've been a musician all of my life. I had played on the Sunset Strip in the 80s with knuckleheads like Warrant and Poison back when the big hair bands ruled the world (this will be salient later in this book).

So, Jimmy asked me what my plan was, and I told him, figuring I had nothing to lose at this point. He listened and then said, "Hang on a minute," and disappeared into the room adjoining his office. I heard him dial his cell phone, mumble a few things to whomever was on the other end, and a minute or so later came back into his office handing me the cell phone.

I looked at him quizzically, like, "What?" He pushed it closer to me as if to say, "Here. Take it." So, I did. I put the phone up to my ear, and disgruntledly said, "Hello?"

The voice on the other end was distinctive. It said, "Hey Andrew, this is Steven Tyler, man. Hey man, listen, ya know, I know what you're going through, man, having second thoughts about the whole treatment thing, y'know. I get it. I mean I was a coke guy too, right? I was sitting right where you're sitting now. I know where you're coming from, man. Listen, y'know, I mean, I realize you don't have your money right now, and y'know, it'll be coming in a few days y'know, so why not maybe just hang out a few days, y'know, at least 'til your money comes, y'know, and then maybe if you're still feeling the same way, then maybe just go then, man!"

I use exclamation points after his sentences because that's just how he talks. "But hey man, listen, in the meantime, do me a favor man, okay? From here on out just be as fucking honest as you can man, okay? Don't hold anything back. I mean, just say whatever you're fucking thinking, alright?! No matter what! Just be as honest as you fucking can! Alright? Promise?"

So, I mumbled something like, "Okay, I suppose so, but just until my money comes." I figured after all; it was Steven Tyler. So, I stuck around out of deference to one of my all-time music idols and never left.

For the next few days I *was* honest — *rigorously* honest with everyone I encountered — patients, nurses, staff — everyone. Frankly, my hope was that I would get kicked out so that I could blame others for my departure. Yet, no matter how brusque or offensive I was, no one rejected me. No one kicked me out. I was being accepted for whom I was despite myself, which was an unfamiliar experience. This made an impact on me, and accounts for my first experiential *aha* insight: that I could be honest and not be rejected. That was a revelation.

The second experiential *aha* that I had in treatment happened when a few days later I found out that Steven Tyler had taken that call from Jimmy at 4 a.m. local time while in Japan. Someone I looked up to felt I was worth helping despite having nothing to offer him. Steven Tyler's selfless act provided experiential evidence that perhaps I had *some* intrinsic value — which disconfirmed my worthless identity at that time.

Experiential interventions, intentional or not, are ten times more powerful than those gained by conversation in talk therapy.

Eventually during that treatment episode I resolved that, if I were truly able to guarantee my behavior, I would probably never need my parents' inheritance money anyway. The idea that I could actually succeed at something, or even realize my potential became plausible. *I began to believe in myself again.*

Jimmy and I are friends and colleagues to this day. At the time of this publication, he is an expert interventionist based out of the Coachella Valley, CA. Although I do interventions, if I had an intervention that I felt exceeded the scope of my expertise, I would have Jimmy handle it without hesitation. His site is: www.weissinterventions.com.

A few years ago I sent Steven a thank-you note through Jimmy upon graduation from the Hazelden Betty Ford Graduate School of Addiction Studies, acknowledging his selfless act of kindness in 2014. I let him know his selfless act would have a positive ripple effect on others' lives. So far, so good.

On a more humorous side note, Jimmy was present when I was discharged from The Betty Ford Center at 12:01 a.m. on the day I was scheduled to go. I wasn't going to wait until morning.

A year or so later, as I was undergoing the stringent admissions process to enter grad school, I approached him about a possible letter of reference. During this visit at his (then) new gig at Northbound Treatment Center in Newport Beach, CA, I asked him, in retrospect, whether at the time I was discharged from Betty Ford he thought that I was going to "make it." He kind of chuckled to himself, looked down, and shook his head. "Nope."

I *love* proving people wrong.

SOCIOPATH OR ADDICT?!

Getting back to my point on values and locus of motivation, going into treatment I was internally motivated, but out of greed and fear. These were values I had adopted out of a need for *congruence* with addictive behaviors that I had been unable to shake over nearly two decades of daily use. Despite the volume of my drug and alcohol consumption, and the fact that I knew something was severely wrong with me, I didn't consider that substance use had anything to do with it.

In fact, a few years before the wheels fell off, I looked myself up in the DSM-V (Diagnostic & Statistical Manual), a book we shrinks use to figure out, *What the hell was that*?! when we run across some obscure set of symptoms in patients. I wanted to figure out what was *wrong* with me. I resigned myself to the possibility I was fundamentally defective. After all, my behavior was like someone without access to their conscience — a sociopath. I had even watched a number of documentaries on criminal sociopaths such as Ted Bundy and Jeffrey Dahmer, and was able to relate to many of the behaviors, mindsets, and attitudes they exhibited both in childhood and adulthood with the exception, of course, of murder.

But that said, according to the DSM-V, among the traits of a sociopath are:

- lack of remorse
- charm
- intelligence
- dishonesty
- manipulativeness
- narcissistic entitlement
- spontaneity
- lack of empathy

It was easy to reach a conclusion of sociopathy without the understanding I now have about addiction. Outwardly, I met all of these criteria; but, one fundamental difference between a sociopath and a person afflicted with addiction is that sociopaths do not experience guilt and shame associated with their behaviors.

Addicts have a functioning conscience despite their best efforts to squelch it. They may not show it, but they feel guilt and shame for their lying, duplicity, and lack of ability to control their behavior. Sadly, the perceived solution to that shame is more addictive behavior(s), which reinforces belief that addicts have no conscience — as evidenced by the ease with which they engage in high risk activities, many criminal in nature.

No one likes a hypocrite. When I Googled *hypocrisy*, the definition that came up is this:

> *The practice of engaging in the same behavior or activity for which one criticizes another or the practice of claiming to have moral standards or beliefs to which one's own behavior does not conform.*

The definition refers to what I call *external hypocrisy*. There is something abhorrent about being shamed for a behavior, and then observing the same behavior, for which we had been condemned, by the same judgmental person.

But what if we are both perpetrators, and critics, of our own offensive behavior?

Internal hypocrisy occurs when addiction-based values are at odds with innate, healthy values. In chronic addiction, this internal discrepancy becomes a source of distress as our egregious, addictive behaviors progressively deviate further and further from our innate values.

As my internal hypocrisy increased with time, ever-greater volumes of substances were required to cope with it. Toward the end of my active use, trips to the hospital for cocaine and alcohol-induced seizures became more frequent. My addiction-fueled behaviors made me an external hypocrite to stakeholders in my life, and an internal hypocrite through betrayal of my innate values.

My double life was literally killing me.

I was engaged in civil war with myself, while desperately attempting to maintain outward appearances with others.

As I gained insight through treatment, I discovered that my innate, healthy values were always present, but were buried by 18 years of chemical and other addictions.

One of the gifts of recovery is an opportunity to consciously *choose* and implement values that will better serve us as we go through the process of imagining an idealized future version of ourselves and the reality to which we aspire. Values that no longer serve our vision get rooted out and discarded, replaced by our innate values and those we aspire to possess.

Starting from scratch, we *design* the person and future we wish to have moving forward from the ground up. In doing so, we can literally become anyone we want.

HOW SHAME WORKS

I like to think of shame as Emotional Cancer. It is insidious, and does tremendous damage, often before being diagnosed. Those not in denial about having shame are usually in denial about the depth of impact of their problem. The feedback loop between shame and addiction eats away at our self-esteem just like termites that undermine the foundation of a house. Left unchecked, the downward spiral continues until we no longer even bother to aspire. We do not *believe* we deserve success or happiness.

THE CABIN STORY

A debilitating shame-based identity along with the inability to imagine successful alternative realities can conspire to produce a deadly mindset. The following story describes one of the lowest points in my life:

> *Approximately 18 months after leaving treatment at The Betty Ford Center, I was up at a cabin in Upper Michigan by myself and I was financially strapped. Since filing for divorce, I had been paying for all of my soon-to-be-ex's living expenses in California while she "couldn't" find work. I was also paying for all of my girlfriend's living expenses in California, while she was presumably working through some legal issues related to the same Xanax that got me into trouble. In addition, I was paying my own living expenses in Wilmington, NC, where my girlfriend had expressed a desire to live so she could get out of the rat race that was Los Angeles.*

> *To make matters worse, the job I had transferred to nearly a year earlier was eliminated just three months after relocating. So, by this time I had spent literally every penny I had to my name, with the exception of just enough gas money to get me from the cabin to the airport for my flight back to North Carolina the next morning. I didn't even have any food in the cabin, so I would not eat until maybe I had some free crackers on the plane.*

> *The final straw was the realization that my girlfriend was probably never going to move from California because she had gone back to using meth — and she was willing to bend her values to acquire it.*

> *I was despondent.*

> *I began looking around the cabin, trying to figure out how to stage my demise so that at least whoever found me wouldn't be horrified and have to clean up a lot.*

My people-pleasing even extended posthumously.

At just that moment, the idea of doing myself in made *perfect* sense.

You see, until then, I had *always* had money. Usually a lot. But I overidentified with it to the extent that I equated it with my value. I truly believed in my heart of hearts that I had no intrinsic value. With no money, I had no value whatsoever. My value was *solely* dependent upon the size of my wallet, which was empty. Of course, this belief was only reinforced by the fact that when the money ran out, so did my girlfriend.

I don't recall exactly how I survived that experience. But I did learn a couple of things that I could have learned no other way. In fact, in retrospect, I consider that half hour or so to have been 100 percent necessary to my recovery. Had it not occurred, I would not have hurt enough to be motivated to change. I never wanted to experience that kind of pain again, nor did I want anyone else to. That experience made me who I am today and taught me:

1. Not everyone left me, so I must have at least *some* intrinsic value.

2. Killing one's self can be a completely logical alternative to living under the wrong circumstances.

So, low self-esteem and viewing no alternative outcomes is quite a deadly combination. The degree to which *doing myself in made perfect sense* is still chilling when I put myself in that memory. It was a cold calculation with a clear solution. I remember it as though it were yesterday, and hope I never forget it.

The good news is that a month later I learned that I had been accepted into the Hazelden Betty Ford Graduate School of Addiction

Studies. I applied everything I learned there toward myself, and have since devoted my energies to ensuring that as few others as possible suffer the pain to which I nearly succumbed.

One method I use to assess shame's damage to patients' self-esteem is to administer the aforementioned *Magic Wand Thought Experiment*. In this exercise, I give them an imaginary magic wand and have them write a detailed vision of how they, and their world, would be if they could have it any way they wanted it.

Patients' difficulty in conjuring an image of reality where their predominant emotion day in and day out is deep gratitude, may be astonishing to the average person; but, as the previous anecdote illustrates, it is not unusual in the population with whom I work.

The *Magic Wand Thought Experiment* exercise provides fertile ground for assessing: the depth of shame afflicting patients; the degree of learned helplessness and hopelessness they are experiencing; and the work necessary to move them toward their true potential. Damage to self-esteem *must* be overcome if we are to reconnect with our True Self and fulfill our potential.

Consistently behaving in a manner aligned with our chosen and innate values, rather than those imposed by addiction, restores self-esteem. Walking in integrity drains the cesspool of resentment that a shame-based personality fills, and banishes shame from our emotional lexicon. Integrity, a Stage Two Recovery feature, is made possible by Stage One abstinence from addictive behaviors.

RESIDUAL SELF-IMAGE

In the movie, *The Matrix*, the main character, Neo, was afflicted with something Morpheus referred to as his residual self-image. Anyone experiencing substantial change has one, regardless of past addiction or not. Our residual self-image is a lagging Identity, which is usually unconscious, and is capable of undermining healthy growth if we are not aware of its presence. Those recovering from addiction always have a residual self-image heavily informed by the shame of their past. Even after years of recovery, we need to be keenly aware of our residual self-image.

The following video is the scene in The Matrix when Neo was enlightened about his residual self-image, and helps us to understand its nature.

 7.1

The late great Earnie Larsen said, "We can never outperform our self-image for long." We need to be acutely aware of our residual self-image as we undergo the change and growth process. It is a lagging attribute.

The way it works is that when we experience a period of rapid growth, we may need to pause until our residual self-image catches up with our improved reality, or at least be aware of the emotional impact of the discrepancy between them.

Discrepancy between our reality and our residual self-image feels *unfamiliar*.

In our habitual state of shame, success feels unfamiliar. Feelings of unfamiliarity are usually interpreted as *wrong*; and so without adequate self-awareness we will find a way to return our circumstances back into something that feels *right*, through self-sabotage. In the absence of self-awareness, our self-image becomes like a thermostat. This will be important later on in UTR, as our reality surpasses that which we feel we deserve.

In the decades leading up to treatment I'd managed to consistently pull the rug out from under myself when progress felt unfamiliar. I went from rural, central Wisconsin to playing in front of 10,000 fans within 18 months. In the big-hair days the Sunset Strip was the place to prove yourself as a musician. After that, I published two separate music magazines — one in Salt Lake City (*Jam Magazine*) and one in Minneapolis (*Encore Magazine*). I was a Series-7 Registered Representative owning a corporate retirement plan consulting firm for 15 years, managing tens of millions of dollars with clients all over the country. I've taught music — have owned and operated a recording studio — I was a mortgage broker — I owned a coffee shop — and even invented an electronic product from scratch. That $160,000 lump of electronics and plastic is now sitting in a bin in my home office (I should probably resurrect that project).

Now I'm a clinician and author. Someone once said I've lived a *Forrest Gump* life. That may not be far from the truth.

But during past periods of growth or success, my self-image was never congruent with the progress I made or the successes I had. The result was a pattern of self-imposed failure following each success. Addictions of various sorts always impaired my self-image throughout those experiences, and over time, the pattern of failure led to deeply-ingrained learned helplessness. After a few decades of this I had all but given up on the idea of a meaningful life. And so I accepted my destiny as a paper-pusher in a dead-end cubicle job, on a cube farm at a large corporation, in backroom operations, for crap hourly wages thinking to myself, *Well, I guess this is it.*

Toward the end, during my last five years in active addiction, I was drinking two bottles of rum a day — doing lines of cocaine at my desk and in the restroom — smoking pot before work, during breaks, at lunch and after work. I made a beeline to my favorite watering hole, Tinhorn Flats in Burbank, after work. My nickname was "3:42 Andrew" — that time being 42 minutes after I clocked out from work. Those last years of my life in addiction were like the movie, *Groundhog Day* — each day being a repeat of the last. That is not living — it is existing.

My life at that time was not reflective of my true potential.

By the time I attended treatment, I had forfeited willingness to aspire. I did not want to disappoint myself nor the stakeholders in my life yet again. To put it another way, I feared both failure *and* success.

One turning point in treatment was when my therapist at The Betty Ford Center, Mike Potter, asked, "Hey Andrew, what do you think you could accomplish if you could just get out of your own way?" This is a practical version of my *Magic Wand Thought Experiment*. It seemed like a compelling question — one that I am still answering.

When we reconnect with our conscience, identify and choose healthy values, and align our daily behavior with them by *walking in integrity,* our residual and current self-image integrate into one, and reflect our new reality. We are on the path to realizing our full potential. As a result, we feel better about who we are, here and now. We don't have to wait for some distant future to be happy because our happiness comes from who we are, not from our circumstances.

To quote Eckhart Tolle:

> *You can only lose something that you have,*
> *but never something that you are.*

Once we go through the one-time Authentication process of recovering our True Self, we become safer to love. We become consistent, and have well-established consciously-chosen values and boundaries, so others do not have to worry about whether we are going to change right out from under them resulting in yet another needless, traumatic relationship breakup. From the position of the

True Self, we are better able to assess the suitability of others for long-term relationships, as well as discern the depth of those relationships and risks we are willing to take.

SUMMARY

STAGE 1 RECOVERY — PREVENT RELAPSE

+ Resentment is *always* a by-product of external motivation. Anyone can abstain from substances for a while using external motivation, but never for very long. Resentment overcomes any good will toward the person or circumstances for whom, or from which, we are abstaining.
+ Shame ensues when we identify with external things — money, socially-imposed status symbols, etc. This is dangerous to recovery because *things* can be taken away, whereas *who we are* cannot.

STAGE 2 RECOVERY — REGAIN AUTHENTICITY

+ According to the ACA *Big Red Book* and UTR, being our True Self is the ideal state of being in the present. Recovery is so-named because that is what we are recovering: our True Self. Authenticity comes from identification with the True Self and its values.
+ ACA meetings provide the most safe and effective forum in which to regain our True Self. As we assert our authenticity in such an environment, the love and acceptance we experience is generalized into the real world, and with wonderful results.
+ We must develop the courage to accept that we may not be everyone's "flavor of the day" as we assert our authenticity. Others either adapt, or rotate out of our lives. Those *others* may be spouses, family members, and even our children. Not everyone we lose is a loss.

STAGE 3 RECOVERY — ENHANCE SPIRITUAL CAPACITY

+ As we change on a fundamental level into our True Self, we experience awe at the contrast between our old, shame-based selves, and our True Self. The love we experience from others on this journey, often for the first time, opens our heart to the possibility of a more reliable, infinite source of love afforded by a higher power.

+ People being human, we may learn there are terms and conditions placed upon others' love. This realization naturally causes us to seek a more reliable source of love, such as that available from a higher power.

+ Being addicts, when we experience love of our True Self from others as a result of authenticity, we wonder where we can get more and better love. Such seeking opens us up to the possibility of a spiritual relationship.

CHAPTER 8

HOW MEDITATION WORKS

MEET THE NEW CEO — YOU

Since self-awareness is the first step in fundamental change, this requires that we develop the capacity to "think about what we are thinking about" — or perhaps it would be more accurate to say "observe what we are thinking about." Only in a state of self-awareness are we able to change what we are thinking about — our thoughts being the sole source of our suffering. After all, we cannot change that of which we are unaware.

The clinical term for self-observation is *meta-cognition*. I only like to say that because it makes me sound really smart. Here it is again: "meta-cognition."

An excellent way to become more self-aware is through the practice of meditation.

Meditation, or mindfulness, is scientifically proven to be useful in emotional self-regulation and in developing the ability to self-reflect. As such, it is considered an evidence-based intervention (in other words, insurance companies will pay for it). It was through leading Intensive Outpatient groups, where meditation is a program requirement, that I became familiar with it. I underwent the process along with my patients; and, meditation turned out to be a great experience even in early stages of the practice (when both the patients and I felt inept at it).

For our purposes, there are three types of meditation with which to become familiar: Practical, Experiential, and Directive.

PRACTICAL MEDITATION

One of the practical ways I have found to begin thinking about what we are thinking about is by subscribing to (and using) the Headspace app: www.Headspace.com. This app has entertaining, informative animations that illustrate the rudimentary principles of meditation. YouTube contains a number of animations from Headspace that provide valuable insight into what meditation is — and is not — as well as how to get started. Here is a link to some of those animations to give you an idea of practical meditation:

 8.1

Among the many positives of this app are:

- Easy to use
- Entertaining, meaningful animations to illustrate concepts
- SHORT meditations — 3-5 minutes
- Effective guided meditations
- It's free for quite a while and easy to unsubscribe
- Many specific areas are covered, depending on your interests — relaxation, productivity, sports, etc.

What are you waiting for? Download it. Recovery is about *doing*. Incorporate Headspace into your daily regimen as frequently as possible at first. There is no down-side to absorbing this material.

EXPERIENTIAL MEDITATION

The goal of Experiential meditation is to adopt the perspective of the *Conscious Observer* of our thoughts. This state provides an *experiential* state of peace previously unknown to those unfamiliar with meditation. It is from this perspective that we may truly contemplate our Identity as a being possessing dual citizenship in both the material and spiritual worlds. It is in this state that we relate and commune with the Universe.

Experiential guided meditation involves shedding layers of awareness in descending order from Environment —> Body —> Thoughts —> Spirit (as in spiritual). We realize that every state besides a *spiritual* one is *environmental*. This brand of meditation results in relaxation, and disengagement from the world. Patients who engage in this type of meditation report feeling somewhat like they did while under the influence of their substance of choice, without the hangover. This makes sense, as with both substances and meditation we become detached from our environment.

Experiential meditation is designed to put us into a state of pure awareness — a timeless, peaceful, formless state devoid of worldly identity. The goal is to *become no one* — an ideal state in which to commune with our higher power and just *be*. This enables us to connect with the unlimited love and peace that has been available to us all along as citizens of the spiritual world. Hopefully this is a state we will crave to occupy when overwhelmed by circumstances in our material world — a healthy addiction!

I enjoy the guided meditations of Mooji. He is great at peeling away levels of awareness, creating a space to become no one and he has a great sense of humor.

Here are some links to his material:

▷ 8.2

One of my favorite guided meditations by Mooji is:

▷ 8.3

DIRECTIVE QUANTUM MEDITATION

Directive meditations used in the UTR clinical model are called Quantum Guided Meditations. Their purpose is functional, combining state of awareness principles while applying *intention*. Those familiar with Law of Attraction principles will be able to relate to this concept. UTR uses this type of meditation for the purpose of telegraphing our vision for an idealized self into the quantum field, ostensibly enabling the Universe or a higher power to conspire in our favor.

A good example of a quantum guided meditation is:

▷ 8.4

Custom guided meditations are available to my private clients by contacting me via the contact form at www.andrewgpierce.com.

There is no reason why these three modes of meditation cannot be practiced concurrently, but a logical progression for beginners would be the order in which they are presented above.

Like any traditional recovery method, the UTR clinical model requires continuity. Whether it's ongoing participation in 12-Step meetings or guided quantum meditations in UTR, continuity over time is essential to long-term success.

The experiential nature of meditation is absolutely critical in developing the capacity to adopt a more spiritual perspective.

SUMMARY

STAGE 1 RECOVERY — PREVENT RELAPSE

+ Meditation allows us to spend time without worldly stressors making it a tool for relapse prevention.
+ As we practice meditation regularly, it becomes apparent that our recovery process may be easier than anticipated, bolstering belief in our ability to succeed in the longer term.

STAGE 2 RECOVERY — REGAIN AUTHENTICITY

+ Meditation, particularly experiential meditation, is a way to access the timeless, immaterial dimension, revealing our True identity as a possessor of dual citizenship.
+ In a state of pure consciousness, we realize that everything — even our thoughts — are *environmental*.
+ As a member of this realm, we identify far more with the Universe than with those things that made us shameful.
+ As a conscious observer of our thoughts and of the world, we immediately experience a change. This peaceful, connected state epitomizes our true, timeless nature — our authentic self.

STAGE 3 RECOVERY — ENHANCE SPIRITUAL CAPACITY

+ The state of being inherent to experiential and directive meditation makes us more comfortable with the concept of divine intelligence. We may, in fact, bask in the exact same state as a higher power, communing with it as our states overlap.

+ In meditation, we intuitively become aware of the possibility of our connection with every other being in the universe.

HOW REALITY WORKS

Part II of this book takes us incrementally through the latest, up-to-the-second scientific paradigms culminating at the edge of our understanding where we may linger — breathing in the same air as the Author of the Universe.

As I drive up to my home after work every day, I press the garage door opener button clipped to my visor, and magically the garage door begins to open. Clearly there is something going on other than magic. What is occurring, in fact, is the button on my remote creates a blip in the electromagnetic field — the same frequency to which my garage door receiver is tuned — resulting in electromagnetic activity vibrating throughout the wires' electromagnetic fields within the garage door opener, et voila! The garage door opens, allowing me to remain dry on wet Florida afternoons.

We take these things for granted these days; but, what we are experiencing is the practical application of our scientific understanding of field theory. The same applies every time we make a cell phone call or send a text to someone thousands of miles away, or in the next room.

CHAPTER 9

HOW SPIRITUAL SKEPTICISM WORKS

As a natural skeptic, I was resistant to the idea of a higher power. Not surprisingly, I have found that there are a number of common themes among most skeptics that need to be resolved before considering a spiritual perspective. Let us briefly explore some of the common barriers to adoption of a world-view containing spirituality.

HOW FAMILY DYSFUNCTION FOSTERS SPIRITUAL SKEPTICISM

I once attended an ACA 12-Step meeting in the Bible belt where the meeting topic was distrust of authority figures. This is an attribute common among those who grew up in dysfunctional families. The subject du jour was how (well-earned) parental distrust becomes generalized to our Higher Power, in this case, a Judeo-Christian God.

The logic of those distrustful of authority figures, particularly God, makes perfect sense.

As a child, who is more god-like than our parents? You may recall Gabor Mate's assertion that the human infant is the most dependent of any creature on the planet (and for the longest period of time). Rejection by a parent presents an existential threat because if the parent abandons the child, the child will literally die as it is unable to fend for itself. A child knows this instinctively.

Many in recovery from substance use disorders grew up in households where they regularly received overt or discreet messages of unacceptability. Many of these children attended church where they learned the consequences of disappointing God, and ascribed the same attributes to God that they did to their parents, as their parents were literally the closest thing to a God existing in their lives. They logically ask, "If my parents could forsake me then why wouldn't an all-important God?"

A cynic would simply infer that if God cared about them, He would not allow dysfunction to occur. The end result is distrust in a higher power.

You may recall from Part I that damage to the insular cortex yields misplaced distrust of the benevolent, and misplaced trust of the untrustworthy. This inverse perspective may well inform many addicts' unwillingness to blindly trust a 12-Step-based Higher Power.

A science-based spiritual model requires no trust. The science underlying UTR has been validated in every experiment ever done to establish or deny its credibility. The UTR practitioner gets to examine every element thereof, so no trust is necessary — certainly not the blind faith that western constructs demand. Furthermore, in UTR, practitioners need only trust themselves, as they are the architects of their lives.

HOW SHAME FOSTERS SPIRITUAL SKEPTICISM

As I said earlier, shame is an emotional cancer. It lends itself to rejection of a higher power in numerous ways. Pathological shame inherent to addiction makes acceptance of a higher power challenging.

- Repression of the True Self in all its forms contributes to a cesspool of shame and unworthiness, giving rise to an unquestioned belief that the afflicted does not deserve happiness, nor the acceptance of a higher power.
- Those in addiction or early recovery tend to possess shame-based personalities, so any religion of which *judgment* is a component intuitively becomes off limits.
- Brené Brown's definition of shame is *unworthiness of connection and love.* Our critical inner voice tells us that God is perfect while we are imperfect, reaffirming our unworthiness.
- A Judeo-Christian God emphasizing forgiveness does not work for us when we feel we are not worthy of forgiveness.
- The Bible portrays both a fire and brimstone God on one hand, and a grace-giving God on the other. These mixed messages discredit the notion of trust in such a God. Faced with mixed interpretations, the ashamed default to the God matching their self-image where fire and brimstone carry the day — a less than desirable scenario for the already-shamed.

A non-judgmental, science-driven higher power informed by Eastern philosophy is easier for shame-based individuals to accept. These disciplines place no conditions for acceptability upon seekers, and proffer a Universe that wants nothing more than for its citizens to live in a state of happiness and fulfillment, while growing into the best possible versions of themselves.

HOW THE FALSE SELF FOSTERS SPIRITUAL SKEPTICISM

Many in early recovery are heavily defended by a False Self put into place as a survival mechanism, often during childhood, to defend against external sources of shame, such as our parents. The greater the shame then, the more heavily-defended we are now. When one has barely a grain of self-worth, any feedback that smacks of rejection is an existential threat. This fear of abandonment goes back to childhood.

Sadly, the False Self in its effort to protect the inner child promotes disconnection — a precursor to the selfsame abandonment it is intended to circumvent. We desperately need love, yet fear-driven unwillingness to be transparent keeps us from connection — human or spiritual.

The battle between vulnerability and love on one hand, and fear and isolation on the other, is an existential battle — truly a hero's journey. The ego denies love in the name of security. After all, the ego asks: *do we want our True Self to risk finding out that it really is unworthy, or would we rather not try, and be able to credibly say it didn't really matter anyway?*

A shame-based individual's ego tells them *it is better to reject than to be rejected.* Our greatest fear is that we are *not* worthy of love and connection. If we don't feel worthy of the grace or benevolence afforded by a higher power, It's safer to reject first. By this logic, believing in a higher power is not worth the risk. Not coincidentally, this is also part of the dynamic behind fear of success: It is better to either sabotage or not try, than to try, and be *proven* a failure.

Yet another barrier to accepting spirituality is rooted in the addict's inability to guarantee their behavior. Performance-based requirements for 'club membership' imposed by many organized religions, and the corresponding judgments that would befall those who fail to conform to said requirements, serve as points of contempt, making engagement in such a religion difficult for the False Self to justify.

Science-based UTR with its bent toward ancient Eastern philosophy circumvents authoritarian aspects inherent to Western religions, resolving barriers thrown up by the False Self while providing the benefits of spirituality.

HOW PROJECTION FOSTERS SPIRITUAL SKEPTICISM

Projection is a clinical term that describes how people avoid dealing with aspects of themselves that they find unacceptable. It is a defense mechanism that manifests in finding fault in others. Disproportionate disgust, anger, indignation, and gossip about others are good indicators of projected defects.

An exercise I often use to illustrate the concept of projection is this:

In a group setting, I have patients take a few moments to think of the most annoying, irritating person they can recall from their lifetime — someone past or present who *really* got, or gets, under their skin. This person could be a childhood enemy, a coworker, a family member — it doesn't matter.

Then, I have them describe in as colorful, yet specific a manner as possible, those aspects of the individual they find abhorrent. Common adjectives include arrogant, condescending, dishonest, dismissive, egotistical, liar, cheater, know-it-all, etc.

Finally, I have each group member share, in some depth, their experiences with these individuals to relive the emotions they elicit.

After everyone is sufficiently indignant, I have them whip out a list they compiled during a recent group session where we went over some aspects they disliked about *themselves* prior to their addictions taking over, or during, or afterward. Without exception, the adjectives used to describe those that they most hated were attributes they possessed and found to be unacceptable.

Projection belies self-hatred. Nearly all of my clients who suffered at the hands of addicted parents report having vowed that they would *never* become like their parents, whom they hold in high contempt. But they have often *become* like their parents.

Turning the indignation and disgust held against our parents toward ourselves is, for many, too painful to bear — thus, projection.

Nonetheless, if we unconsciously know that we are just like the people we despise most, then we inevitably believe we deserve the same eternal condemnation we would wish upon them.

If A is us, B is our parents, and C is condemnation by God, our logic follows this simple high school algebra axiom:

If A = B, and B = C, then A = C

In English, if we are like our parents, and our parents deserve condemnation because of their abhorrent character attributes, then *we* must deserve condemnation. This is not exactly a formula for embracing spirituality.

Projection adds a layer of pathology, a smokescreen imposed by the False Self, to protect us from what we believe in our heart of hearts to be true about ourselves — that we do not deserve the consideration of a higher power. Projection keeps us from accepting the fact that we probably need the grace and alliance of a loving higher power in our lives, but serves as a barrier to this spiritual resource.

SUMMARY

STAGE 1 RECOVERY — PREVENT RELAPSE

+ Projection delays our ability to face our self-loathing, and denies us access to the pain that would normally push us toward the grace available in a benevolent higher power. Identifying and resolving projection enables us to accept a spiritual intervention — decreasing stress, and thus, relapse potential.

+ Replacing the False Self with authenticity enables us to connect with others — lack of connection being a primary relapse trigger for those in early recovery.

STAGE 2 RECOVERY — REGAIN AUTHENTICITY

+ As humans we are masterful at adaptation. To survive dysfunctional family members and the world, many of us created a False Self based on our belief that our True Self was unlovable. This shame-based, inauthentic, dishonest False Self perpetuates shame and must be dismantled to make room for the True Self to be shown, and thus, loved.

STAGE 3 RECOVERY — ENHANCE SPIRITUAL CAPACITY

+ The false-self-imposed prison is devoid of intimacy and true love. Built and reinforced from childhood through adulthood, it destroys the possibility of trust in others, as well as trust in a higher power.

+ Distrust disconnects us from the possibility of reaping the benefits afforded by spirituality; and as such, it must be overcome by strategic assertiveness of the True Self, either in mutual support groups or in a therapeutic setting.

+ When we overcome shame, dismantle the False Self, and resolve projection, we increase our capacity to accept a higher power, which eventually displaces shame and the need for defense mechanisms.

CHAPTER 10

HOW LEARNED HELPLESSNESS WORKS

As addicts we often believe that our past will determine our future. Our inability to guarantee our behavior causes us to misjudge our future prospects. This is because our assessment is over-informed by a *past* inability to change — sometimes over the course of many decades-worth of efforts to change. We have learned how to be helpless and we need to learn self-efficacy — the belief that we can change our behavior.

If we do not become a different person than the person who created our past, then we cannot expect our future to differ much from our past. While it is true that in our past we failed at changing into the kind of person who can guarantee their behavior, we also didn't have access to the information about the nature of reality contained in this book. AND — we have huge blind spots in our understanding of ourselves!

Imagine being a blind person who has never flown a plane before trying to fly a jumbo jet from Miami to Hawaii!

That was us. But that was *then*.

The following video is a compilation of salient points from one of the very first lectures presented in this book by Dr. Joe Dispenza. His change model uses many of the same principles we have touched on. The main point here is that we cannot expect to make long-lasting fundamental change as the same person who created our current reality. Although in this video he makes many profound observations, our focus is on the fact that we cannot expect to experience a new personal reality as the same personality. He states, "We must literally become someone else." And he is right.

 10.1

BABY ELEPHANTS

There is a small abstract elephant statue on my desk — a gift from my life-long buddy Tom Larson — which people inevitably ask about. Many presume it is the proverbial "elephant in the room," representing their addiction itself. In many cases, this is a suitable analogy. Others, (half) jokingly, guess that it represents their codependent loved ones' unfaltering memory of past transgressions.

The fact is, it represents learned helplessness.

We have probably all seen the familiar painting of a giant circus elephant munching hay outside of a big-top tent, perhaps between shows, with its rear leg tied to one end of a rope and a stake driven into the ground on the other end. Looking at the picture, we surmise that the full-sized elephant could easily pull the stake out of the ground and go about marauding through the tent or nearby parking lot — but it does not.

Why? Because the elephant has presumably worked for the fair since it was just a baby elephant, at which age the rope and stake were sufficient to keep it from wandering off.

Before long, the baby elephant learned it was unable to break free from its tether — and quit trying.

Learned helplessness.

The rope, stake, and their power over the now-adult elephant, have become sufficient to keep the grown elephant from *trying* to break free.

So, it is with addiction and recovery. If we don't believe we can succeed, we will not try.

In 2004, while in the depths of my addiction(s), I was unable to imagine the possibility of regaining control of my addictive behaviors. I was in a tailspin. I eventually saw the writing on the wall, and resigned myself to the fact that I would never be able to refrain from spending on my addictions faster than I was able to earn what they cost. Seeing no prospects for changing my trajectory, and not wanting to drag my family down with the ship, I resolved to divorce my first wife, leaving both she and my children a financial life raft in the form of the mansion in which we lived (which was paid-for), and sufficient assets to see the children through high school and college. I framed this to myself and anyone who would listen as a selfless act.

My hope back then was to die in a substance-induced fog — preferably in a sudden and painless manner such as a one-vehicle car accident. For whatever reason, I never had the guts to make this happen, despite eyeing numerous telephone poles. So the dying part never worked out; but, my daughter hasn't spoken to me in 16 years as of this writing, so in some ways I did die.

The point here is that many in addiction or early recovery are incapable of even conjuring an image of what a life without substances would look like. They have learned how to be helpless.

One way I measure learned helplessness in new patients is to administer the *Magic Wand Thought Experiment* mentioned briefly in Part I and explained here:

10.2

In this assignment, I tell the patient I am handing them a magic wand with which they may make their future look ***any*** *way they want it to*, with *no* restrictions whatsoever (it *is* a magic wand, after all, right?)

I ask them to write an essay describing their idealized world, and how they would *be* as fully-realized individuals.

Despite their best efforts, a vast majority are unable to imagine such a world with any clarity — a fact they find alarming. This is relevant because it illustrates how insidious their addiction has become over time — depriving them of their ability to even *imagine* possibilities.

Common responses when processing the assignment at their next session range from, "Well, I wanted to be realistic." to "What does this have to do with anything?!" to "I don't understand the question." These responses reveal learned helplessness, and the patients' depth of disbelief in a higher power's ability to intervene on their behalf.

HOW LIFE IS LIKE A PROSPECTUS

Stockbrokers are required to include the caveat: "Past Performance Does Not Guarantee Future Results" when touting prospective investments. People in recovery need to reflect on this when pondering their future prospects. In the investment context, the sentence is intended as a warning. In my patients' context, it is intended to instill hope while raising awareness that their future has nothing to do with their past. UTR resolves the skepticism of low self-efficacy by way of one of its core components — quantum mechanics — which is *all* about possibility and inherent uncertainty.

> *Once you learn quantum mechanics,*
> *you are never really the same again.*
> —Fabric of the Cosmos

When we truly understand the nature of quantum mechanics and reality, we are (and probably should be) surprised that the *only* thing keeping us the same person we were two seconds ago, yesterday, or five years ago is our *memory* of whom we are *supposed* to be — our identity — reinforced by our familiar surroundings. Period. Our beliefs about *who we are supposed to be* are literally the only things constraining us from being — well, any*thing* and any*one* — imaginable. We just don't *know* this.

In UTR, we practice *forgetting* our identity, making it possible to imagine with far greater clarity a future with no limitations.

A skeptic's intellect tends to work against them. Trusting a power greater than themselves, when self-reliance and intellect have served them so well in the past, seems an unnecessary risk. Twelve-step programs ask those in addiction aspiring to recover, to ". . . turn our will and our lives over to the care of God as we understand Him." At such times, "We stood at the turning point . . ." and until now, always turned back.

Joe Dispenza's *Rewired* series on Amazon Prime Video does an excellent job addressing the *analytical* barrier to change (Episode 2). The series also provides a cursory overview of his change model that heavily informs the UTR change model administered to patients in my individual practice and seminars. Please watch the first four episodes of the series.

 10.3

The series provides a glimpse of many of the principles I use with patients in my practice — particularly field theory and meditation aspects.

What we believe to be true about ourselves and our world informs our ability to change. As skeptics, we do not buy into things we do not understand. Belief that we can change is fundamental to our ability to change. The principles laid out in the *Rewired* series serve as a strong basis for belief that we can change.

SUMMARY

STAGE 1 RECOVERY — PREVENT RELAPSE

+ Overcoming learned helplessness relating to our addictions gives us an attitude of hope and possibility that removes fuel for relapse as we refocus on fulfilling our potential rather than the past.
+ Past performance does not guarantee future results.
+ Baby elephants learn early on that they cannot escape a small rope wrapped around a stake in the ground. Those in addiction have, likewise, convinced themselves they cannot quit using them, even though they can, and without as much difficulty as they imagine. Realizing this is critical for those afraid to even imagine what a life in recovery could be like.
+ The *Magic Wand Thought Experiment* exposes the depth of learned helplessness of someone considering recovery.

STAGE 2 RECOVERY — REGAIN AUTHENTICITY

+ We put ourselves first, possibly for the first time, we learn what we truly want, what we aspire to, and we resume dreaming our forgotten dreams.

+ In our most authentic state, our choices and behaviors reflect our true values — a dynamic that differs greatly from the False Self. We do not live in a vacuum so when we change, those around us, as well as our circumstances, change more to our liking.

+ The *Magic Wand Thought Experiment* forces us to remember who we wanted to be before learned helplessness cast its spell on us. Getting back in touch with our true purpose feels authentic, and provides internal motivation to live up to our true potential.

STAGE 3 RECOVERY — ENHANCE SPIRITUAL CAPACITY

+ We are not a bunch of subatomic particles. We are energy with a consciousness. Understanding this, we are able to ponder a more spiritual perspective.

+ When we overcome the learned helplessness that bound us to our old addictive attitudes and behaviors, such fundamental change enables us to consider the possibility of further change in the form of harnessing spirituality.

+ The *Magic Wand Thought Experiment*, and subsequent processing in a therapeutic setting, gets us back in touch with our true aspirations, and reminds us of how effortless life was at those times in our lives when we were our True Selves, enabling us the benefit of 20/20 hindsight to see how the Universe conspired in our favor at those times.

HOW *NOTHING* WORKS

We must drill down from the macro-world of our daily existence, *through* the micro-world, into the very fabric of reality itself . . . and then apply the new insights gained to our macro-world.

HONEY, I SHRUNK THE UNIVERSE!

Everything around us is made up of atoms. If you recall your high school physics class you know atoms have quite a bit of empty space between their component subatomic particles. In fact, 99.999999 percent of atoms, and thus all of the matter around us, is empty space. That's a *lot* of empty space in relation to material substance. Let us put this into perspective.

- Only .0000001 percent of the universe is material — stars, galaxies, people, paper-towel holders, etc.
- If you removed the empty space from every human being on the planet, you would end up with an object smaller than a sugar cube.

- To put it another way, if you removed the empty space from between all of the subatomic particles comprising all of the concrete and steel in the Empire State Building, you would be left with something the size of a tiny grain of rice.
- If you blew up the nucleus of, say, a helium atom to the size of a marble, its electron's orbit would exceed the circumference of a pro football stadium.

Everything that is *not* material — in other words, the other 99.999999 percent of the universe — is *field*-energy. Turns out all that seemingly empty space between atoms' subatomic particles is not empty.

In *Breaking the Habit of Being Yourself*, Joe Dispenza discusses the implications of this reality to assert his concept of a divine intelligence:

> *I hope by now you agree on some basic underlying concepts of the quantum model — that all physical reality is primarily energy existing in a vast web that is interconnected across space and time. That web, the quantum field, holds all probabilities, which we can collapse into reality through our thoughts (consciousness), observation, feelings, and state of being.*
>
> *But is reality nothing but indifferent electromagnetic forces acting on and in response to one another? Is the animating spirit within us simply a function of biology and randomness? I've had conversations with people who hold this view. Ultimately the discussion leads to a dialogue that goes something like this:*
>
> *Q: Where does the intelligence that keeps our heart beating come from?*
> *A: That's a part of the autonomic nervous system.*

Q: Where is that system located?

A: The brain. The brain's limbic system is part of the autonomic nervous system.

Q: And within the brain, are there specific tissues that are responsible for keeping the heart beating?

A: Yes.

Q: What are those tissues made up of?

A: Cells.

Q: And what are those cells made up of?

A: Molecules.

Q: What are those molecules made up of?

A: Atoms.

Q: And what are those atoms made up of?

A: Subatomic particles.

Q: And what are those subatomic particles primarily composed of?

A: Energy.

> *When we arrive at the conclusion that our physiological vehicle is made up of the same stuff as the rest of the universe, and these folks bump up against the notion that what animates the body is a form of energy — the same 99.999999 percent "nothing" that constitutes the physical universe — they either shrug and walk away or come to realize that there is something to this notion that a unifying principle pervades all of physical reality.*

> *Isn't it ironic, then, that we keep all of our attention on the 0.000001 percent of reality that is physical? Are we missing something? If this "nothing" consists of energy waves that carry*

information, and this force organizes our physical structures and their functioning, then it certainly makes sense to refer to the quantum field as an invisible intelligence. And since energy is at the basis of all physical reality, that intelligence I've just described to you has organized itself into matter.

Think of the preceding conversation as a kind of template for how this intelligence has constructed reality. The quantum field is invisible potential energy that is able to organize itself from energy to subatomic particles to atoms to molecules, and on up the line to everything. From a physiological perspective, it organizes molecules into cells into tissues into organs into systems, and finally into the body as a whole. Put another way, this potential energy lowers itself as a frequency of wave patterns until it appears as solid.

It is this universal intelligence that gives life to that field and everything in it, including you and me. This power is the same universal mind that animates every aspect of the material universe. This intelligence keeps our hearts beating, and our stomachs digesting food, and oversees an incalculable number of chemical reactions per second that take place in every cell. Moreover, the same consciousness prompts trees to grow fruit and causes distant galaxies to form and collapse.

My initial reading of this passage caused me to further explore the assertion of a Divine Intelligence, realizing I couldn't simply take his word for it. The ensuing research, contained in the remainder of this book, yielded the spiritual basis of the UTR change model.

HOW EMPTY SPACE WORKS

So, what, then, *is* that 99.999999 percent of space between atoms' component parts?

The following brief video shows *empty* space. It is incredible, factual, and we see how this concept is critical to our understanding of how spirituality, and many of its aspects, works.

 11.1

There is no need to become fixated on the details in the video. For now, take away the fact that there is literally *no such thing* as empty space. In fact, it is packed with at least 17 immaterial *fields*, which we will explore in detail later. If the universe were a painting, these fields would be the three-dimensional canvas upon which the world — everything we see and everything we don't — is painted.

Exactly how pervasive are these fields?

Consider for a moment the letters that make up the words on the pages of this book. The letters are actually made up of microscopic dots of ink molecules sprayed onto the pages of the paper that is composed of paper molecules, *all* of which are composed of atoms that, in turn, consist of subatomic particles. Each subatomic particle is derivative of "perturbations" in one of three respective fields from which everything we see originates (more on that later).

The letters, words, sentences, and ink on the page are being perceived by your brain. Your brain is derivative of the same subatomic particles and field perturbations as is the content and media comprising this book. The neurons that synthesized the ideas contained herein (those in my mind or brain) are derivative of the selfsame fields that comprise you, the book, ink, etc.

This is a closed system consisting of author (me), content, media (paper, computer, etc.) by which the information is conveyed, and reader (you), all of which are derivative of the same continuous fields. Given this, one could ask, "Why not just leave out the middleman?! Why is a book even needed? This information was always present within the fields, so why don't I just know all of this stuff like the author does?" To put it in more scientific terms, the fields need not have organized themselves into subatomic particles comprising neurons in my brain, which all fired in such a manner that I ultimately came up with the content of this book.

Remember, my brain and its neurons are derivative of the exact same fields that your brain is! Throughout the entire "author-content-reader" system, the quantum fields are *the* common denominator permeating the subjective reader (you), the subjective author (me), and the objective media by which this information is being conveyed from my brain to yours.

The medium through which this information is transmitted is derivative of the same fields as the source and receiver of the information, whether via electronic screen, paper, or by voice through the air, which is also derivative of — you guessed it — the quantum fields.

We are all inextricably connected by the fields, of and through which we and everything in the universe exists.

The fields are continuous, indivisible, and are the fundamental element(s) upon which *all* of reality is built. All realities, to be more precise. But more on that later.

By the way, a perturbation is a small disturbance in a field that constitutes the means by which a subatomic particle comes into material existence. It literally goes from an energy (field) state, into a material (particle) state by virtue of a precise electromagnetic charge (perturbation), occurring at a very specific point within that particle's field, and then interacting with the Higgs Field. This concept will be fully fleshed out later in the book with visuals to make it much easier to understand.

HOW THE TRUE SELF WORKS

The earliest phases of the UTR clinical track introduce the concept of an idealized version of ourselves in the form of the *Magic Wand Thought Experiment*. This acts as a beacon on the horizon toward which we aspire to move as we work our way toward the realization of our full potential. Authenticity is a necessary ingredient in identifying our true aspirations and in gaining access to the ability to effectively commune with the Universe; but this wasn't my idea.

It turns out a relationship between our Authentic Self or True Self and the Universe was recognized thousands of years ago by **all** cultures on the planet, independently of each other — no small coincidence. Back then there was no internet or ability to communicate across oceans, so it must be inferred that the importance of the relationship between our true selves and the Universe is a human condition, not specific to any particular culture. The story behind this phenomenon, along with some other profound distinctions, is articulated in the following documentary entitled, *Finding Joe*.

 11.2

Among many gems, one theme explored in the documentary is that when we are authentic, there is no such thing as coincidence. When we recover our authentic state, align our heads and hearts, and mobilize our spiritual connection with the Universe, life becomes effortless as the Universe conspires in our favor. Or, as one of the interviewees in the documentary puts it, "When you truly step forth and trust your bliss, unseen forces have the power to rearrange things to accommodate your step of faith."

The *Finding Joe* documentary was instrumental for me in connecting ancient Eastern philosophy with up-to-the-second quantum field theory — both major features in the UTR change-model used in my practice. Although the documentary makes a strong intuitive argument, I needed to know *how* this worked, which is what the rest of this book is about.

SUMMARY

STAGE 1 RECOVERY — PREVENT RELAPSE

+ The moment we take a step of faith to recover our True Self, the Universe is activated. We begin to notice that it is doing things for us that we could never have orchestrated ourselves.

+ Living in a newly authentic state bolsters belief that we can not only change ourselves, but as a result, our circumstances. We realize that we need not affect all (or any) outcomes through overt effort, and stress decreases. Decreased stress always translates to increased resilience against relapse.

+ Once we overcome the short-term adjustment of others to our True Self, life becomes effortless as we leverage the quantum field, conspiring with a higher power that has become available to us through meditation. This sense of effortless flow decreases stress and thus relapse potential.

+ Connection with a higher power, through repetition and experiencing feedback, increases into faith over time, decreasing stress and fuel for relapse.

STAGE 2 RECOVERY — REGAIN AUTHENTICITY

+ Authenticity is not a new concept. It is prevalent in ancient Eastern philosophy. It is important to self-esteem, and in a state as our True Self, we are best able to leverage the Universe's mechanics to realize our full potential, thus maximizing our happiness.

+ The value of the True Self is likened to a golden Buddha in an ancient Eastern parable referenced in *Finding Joe*.

+ Dispenza posits that the True Self is the most effective transmitter and receiver whereby we leverage the quantum field to mobilize the Universe's mechanics to our benefit.

+ We are 99.999999 percent energy. Coordinating our heads and our hearts into a congruent energy field enables us to not only commune effectively with the Universe, but also with others in an authentic manner, which facilitates the experience of true love — the most wonderful experience we can have in life.

STAGE 3 RECOVERY — ENHANCE SPIRITUAL CAPACITY

+ Understanding that we are 99.999999 percent more empty space than material being reminds us that we are not simply the sum of our material parts (subatomic particles). This insight sets us up to consider the plausibility of *dual citizenship* between the energy and material worlds, and its value.

+ There is a direct correlation between authenticity's congruent energy, and the Universe's responsiveness to its aspirations. This common theme permeates time and space — independently deduced by cultures around the world over the ages who had no ability to communicate with each other.

+ As we gain experience connecting with others' energy, we begin to consider the possibility of connecting with a higher power, and its benefits.

CHAPTER 12

HOW QUANTUM MECHANICS WORKS

It is imperative to gain some fundamental understanding of the quantum nature of the Universe in order to fully participate in UTR practices. Despite not being taught with sufficient rigor in high school physics classes, quantum mechanics has slowly become the predominant paradigm for explaining reality.

The NOVA series, *The Fabric of The Cosmos,* was instrumental in my ability to embrace a worldview based upon a quantum model of reality. The content in the links below serve as a foundation for understanding the counterintuitive nature of reality. Science since then has built upon the foundation of reality covered in the series; and, it is 100 percent relevant to our work. Please watch them all, being mindful that you need not memorize any of the material. The graphics are great at illustrating the presented concepts:

▷ 12.1 – 12.4

The purpose in having you review these NOVA episodes is to turn your perception of reality and the world upside down. The content should spark you to question everything you thought you knew about . . . everything. From this vantage point we are able to be more receptive to radical change and possibility.

One practical application of the now-famous (to physicists and nerds like me) double-slit experiment — which demonstrates that subatomic particles exist in energy (wave) form until *observed by a conscious observer* — is that patients who fully internalize this concept, gain the ability to change far faster those using traditional recovery methods.

The last decade has provided some monumental discoveries in physics. For example, the final piece of the quantum field theory puzzle was put into place in 2012, when the Large Hadron Collider (LHC), built by the European Organization for Nuclear Research (CERN), located near Geneva, Switzerland, proved the existence of the Higgs Field. This demonstrated the mechanism by which energy is converted into matter — super-important stuff in the physics world. The following link best explains what the LHC is, and how it works.

12.5

Now that we have hopefully eviscerated our traditional world view with *Fabric of the Cosmos*, let us build from there.

A hundred years ago, atoms were thought to be the most fundamental building blocks of the universe. Then we found that atoms were composed of subatomic particles — protons, neutrons, and electrons, which we then proclaimed to be fundamental. Then, as technology improved we learned that the protons and neutrons, which comprise the nucleus of most atoms, are made up of even smaller components called quarks: "up" quarks, and "down" quarks, each delineated by its respective "spin," no less. So these subatomic particles were then considered to be the components most fundamental to nature. This physical model for reality — particle physics — was the best working theory we had for many decades.

But particle physics was still flawed and incomplete, leaving too many unanswered questions:

- Where do the particles come from?
- Where do they go?
- Why do they come and go?
- Why do they not fly off willy-nilly, but rather form into atoms?
- Why do they behave the way that they do?
- How do they maintain a relationship with each other, even when separated by huge distances?
- What is in the space separating them from each other?
- How can entangled particles communicate with each other faster than light — instantaneously?
- How does gravity work?

According to Newtonian physics (and Einstein concurred), material objects need to be in direct proximity in order to affect each other — directly or vicariously touching. But subatomic particles simply do not follow these rules. For example, quantum entanglement, as it is called — or what Einstein referred to as "spooky action at a distance" — was inexplicable by traditional Newtonian models.

As pointed out in the *Fabric of the Cosmos* documentary, quantum entanglement occurs when subatomic particles are split. Their behavior defies all Newtonian conceptions of how objects at any distance interact with each other. Entangled particles are essentially tethered together permanently, such that, observing the state of one *simultaneously* impacts the state of the other. Now, according to Einstein, this is impossible for any number of reasons, not the least of which is that according to his calculations, nothing may travel faster than the speed of light. Yet, in all experiments with entangled particles, regardless of their distance from each other, they show *simultaneous* change in state. Quantum entanglement will be much more fully dissected later, as it is critical to UTR.

With insights that defied the conventional wisdom of Einstein and other physicists, it became clear that either more information was required, or that physicists had to start from scratch. Physicists knew they had to keep working on these problems, and they have made considerable progress.

A BRIEF DIVERSION ON TIME AND TIMELESSNESS

One idea central to the UTR change model is that our childhood and adult aspirations are *future memories*. The *Fabric of the Cosmos:* 'Time' episode touches indirectly on how this would work — but is inadequate in that it only shows one possible timeline. Richard Feynman's Infinite Paths model, which we'll go into later, shows that at any given time, *all* possible realities exist concurrently. To put it more simply, there is no possible reality that does not exist at every given point in time.

So in at least *one* of those infinite possible realities, a completely realized, congruent version of yourself is broadcasting a really strong energy signature into the quantum field to which our *current* self is uniquely attuned. If you recall the *Rewired* series, you will remember the fact that we all have a *unique* electromagnetic, or energy signature. Dispenza asserts that its strongest, most congruent form is our True Self in the present. Quantum entanglement enables us to connect between Us-Now and Us-Then. This is possible because in (quantum) reality, time is *not* unidirectional as we see illustrated in the links below:

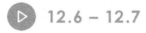

One of the implications of the Delayed-Choice, Quantum Eraser Experiment is that our present affects our past — and our future can affect our present and past — across the various, infinitely possible realities.

TIME TO CONNECT SOME DOTS

The concepts of Quantum Entanglement *plus* Richard Feynman's Infinite Quantum Paths model, which we will explore in Chapter 1, are the basis for Dispenza's contention that an idealized future version of ourselves can, and does, exist. This is not a theoretical abstraction. It's a mathematical certainty. The fuzzy nature of *now* provides the means by which we get there.

Our vision for an idealized future self as outlined in the *Magic Wand Thought Experiment*, reflects the reality in which our idealized self already exists. The process of recovering our authenticity in the present, enhances our ability to *tune in* with greater receptive capability to the vision toward which we are being drawn. Our idealized reality is our 100 percent authentic True Self functioning in our perfect vision of reality. With ongoing meditation practice, we are able to merge our current timeline into that of our idealized self and reality.

In simpler terms, the more congruent and authentic we are in the present, the greater our electromagnetic signature in the quantum field; and thus, the greater our ability to broadcast and receive the electromagnetic signature of entangled, idealized versions of ourselves. A strong unique electromagnetic signature is a *tether* between our current self and our aspirational self.

The ancient Eastern philosophers referenced in *Finding Joe* would assert that there is more at play here. They posit that in our authenticity, the Universe, or our Higher Power, is *listening* as we tune into that idealized future version of ourselves. In this sense, **aspiration while in a state of Authenticity is the strongest form of prayer**. As the Universe is listening, small steps of faith, such as engaging in focused meditation on our aspirational self and reality, are rewarded with material feedback that tells us we are on the right path. This feedback prompts us to continue with our meditative practice, which in turn, provides even more feedback, thus *experientially* reinforcing our faith in the process and our Higher Power. This bilateral dynamic between us, and the Universe, exemplifies the reality and value of our dual citizenship.

DUAL CITIZENSHIP AT WORK

I will share a few examples of my own experiences with this dynamic. One of them suggests that the Universe has a bit of a sense of humor.

Within three weeks of deciding to put together this book, I ran across two individuals who had advanced degrees in theoretical physics. One was a friend of a client for whom I happened to be doing some clinical work in another state. A friend of his had been invited to stay with him for a few days long before I had even conceived of this project. Yet, just as I had put together a skeleton of what I was proposing, this theoretical physicist showed up; and, he and I spent a couple of hours bouncing ideas off of each other. I sought push-back — preferably anything to tell me I was way off base — potentially saving me a year or more of fruitless research. Yet, for better or worse, he agreed that it was a sound idea.

A few weeks later, while back in Florida, I went to get lunch with an old friend, John Henderlite, who had been my counselor at a halfway house in St. Paul, MN, back when I was 17 years old. At lunch I told him about this new idea I was working on for a clinical model and he said, "Hey, my friend is coming down next week to go golfing and he's a retired nuclear physicist. Maybe we could grab a bite together at Joey's on Marco Island for some pizza." I agreed, and sure enough, I ran my idea past him, again, hoping he would push back, so I could either give up, or shore up any weak spots in my model.

He, too, felt it was solid.

We could easily mark these intersections with subject matter experts down to coincidence. One theoretical physicist, perhaps. But two, and at exactly the right time? I've been on the planet for 56 years (at the time of this writing), and have never encountered even *one* theoretical or nuclear physicist.

I chose to interpret the coincidence as feedback from the Universe that maybe I was onto something.

A more subtle, but humorous, example occurred when I flew up to Minnesota to run my then-developing manuscript past my dear friend and colleague Dan Frigo, who was one of my professors (and a former Dean) at the Hazelden Betty Ford Graduate School of Addiction Studies. Dan has considerable expertise, both academically and experientially, in Eastern spiritual philosophy and, of course, addiction. I love and respect Dan as a clinician, friend, and mentor. He has probably forgotten more than I'll ever know.

I was nervous about this meeting because by the time of that pow-wow I had become rather committed to the project, and knew he would be honest.

When we met at the coffee shop in Lindstrom, MN, just down the road from Hazelden, I could tell that Dan had actually read the manuscript, which made me even more nervous. But to my relief and delight, he liked it, further validating the path I was on while providing additional feedback and ideas.

A wonderful and funny synchronicity on this trip was that the first four letters on my rental car's license plate were EMC^2, followed by the month and year of the visit! Of course, physics nerds know that this is an equation from Einstein's Special Theory of Relativity, E=MC squared, defining the relationship between energy and mass.

Once again, this quirky experience could have been coincidence; but, I chose to interpret it as a humorous wink from the Universe that I was on the right track.

When I finally became committed to completing this project, I felt a sense of peace and conviction about seeing it through to its conclusion. My head and heart were aligned. I meditated about it in the UTR-prescribed manner, and things just kept falling into place as I persisted.

NOW IT'S GETTING WEIRD

Another example of this serendipity occurred when I was nearly finished with (or so I thought) the manuscript for this book and decided I'd better figure out the whole publishing aspect of the project. After all, I reasoned, a book isn't going to have a significant impact unless it's published.

Since this is the first book I've written, I knew nothing about publishing. That being the case, I threw a dart at the internet to see what came up. I punched in a few search terms to get some idea of the process. One thing I found out fairly quickly was that some 90 percent of books published engage the services of a literary agent to shop manuscripts around — an idea I wasn't averse to if that's how things get done.

I also did a little research on self-publishing via Amazon, as well as the Hazelden Publishing submission process, those being my initial potential channels. My heart sank when I learned how long it takes (years) from the time of submission to publication with a standard publishing house such as Hazelden Publishing; and furthermore, that I would probably have little editing input once they took over the manuscript.

Finally I figured I would search for literary agents in Florida, resigning myself to the likelihood that any reputable agencies would be on the east coast (Miami) area. Predictably, most of the red dots that appeared on the map of results were over in the greater Miami area.

There was one dot, however, on my side of Florida in Bonita Springs, just up the road (they have since moved to Naples, FL). So, at the very least I thought I might as well pick their brain about publishing to facilitate my research.

I reached out to them by email, and they quickly sent me an e-brochure describing the various publishing options including: self-publishing, vanity publishing, traditional publishing, and something in between called concierge publishing, which is what they do, enabling an author to have as much, or as little help as they want.

I made an appointment and a few days later I met with them.

Turns out the owner, with whom I met, gets the recovery thing, *and* publishes a lot of books with a spiritual angle — exactly the scope and bent of my manuscript. And she liked the concept.

Then I met the head editor; and it turns out, she is well-acquainted with the recovery field *and* has experience in Eastern spirituality modalities. So they *got* the content — *got* what I was trying to accomplish — and were on board with every aspect of the project. And they're right down the street. What are the odds, right?

Again, I could mark it all down to coincidence, but this was getting ridiculously coincidental.

There is more.

I'm one guy. I run a thriving, individual, clinical practice. My schedule is fluid due to people scheduling, cancelling, re-scheduling, etc. Some weeks are balls-to-the-wall. Others can be sparse, depending on what's going on with my patients.

During times when I have needed big blocks of time to write or edit — my clinical schedule has lightened up. When the ball has been in the editor's court — my schedule has filled up.

Furthermore, during the writing and editing phases of this book, challenges presented by patients paralleled themes I was developing — prompting the crystallization of numerous key insights that would otherwise not have come into fruition within these pages had my clients not had coinciding issues.

THE PRACTICAL BENEFITS OF DUAL CITIZENSHIP

To the extent that I have practiced the principles presented in this book, I have clearly received experiential feedback from the Universe — often to the point that it feels a little spooky. In fact, when I practice consistently, things tend to go *so* well that it takes some time for my residual self-image to catch up to my reality. My old, shame-based self, for instance, begins to question whether I can handle the success that comes with co-authoring my ideal reality with a seemingly motivated higher power. But this is what putting the Universe to work for us looks and feels like. It takes some getting used to; but with time, we learn to embrace the unexpected. We become comfortable in the unknown, and in fact, revel in it.

The original purpose of engaging in this process was to reap some of the benefits afforded by spirituality. These consistent experiences reinforce my belief in the importance and value of our dual citizenship as both material and spiritual beings.

The process of testing and using the clinical UTR model, and writing this book, has provided me the following benefits:

- *Hope* for my future has blossomed.
- I've developed *belief* that:
    The Universe is *listening*
    The Universe *cares*
    The Universe wants me to follow my bliss
- I have gained tremendous confidence in pursuing my ambitions.
- My self-esteem has sky-rocketed.
- I am more fearless.
- I have gained confidence in the veracity of my UTR clinical model.
- I believe that others' perceptions about me and my work are positively influenced by the Universe.

As a person in long-term recovery from addiction, but also a spiritual skeptic, these were all unfamiliar experiences for me. But since we are all on the same recovery journey, there is every reason to believe that those who mirror these practices will derive the same benefits. In fact, they *have*. I know this because I have refined and implemented my clinical model with dozens of patients with similar results.

AUTHENTICITY + QUANTUM REALITY = HOPE

Physicists fluent in field theory assert that the quantum fields contain all possible realities at all times, making it possible to *select* a reality that corresponds with our idealized self and world. This is not just a possibility, it is a mathematically proven fact.

When a patient recovers a connection with his or her True Self, they are more easily able to visualize an idealized version of themselves, and the ideal reality in which they aspire to reside. I believe that most in early recovery from addiction have *forgotten* who they are. The *Magic Wand Thought Experiment* reveals deficits in their connection to their authenticity — their congruence with whom they truly are.

How can you know what you want if you don't know who you are?

An idealized version of ourselves already exists here and now — in the form of our True Self. It just happens to be a 3-year-old self that has some growing to do — but we do that work in therapy and in ACA groups. Our reality may need some work, but that's secondary — and besides, it is the one factor over which we have the least influence. Not so with our Inner Child. That ideal version of ourselves is inside of us right now. Point a little bit below your chest. He or she is right there, buried by years of repression and self-denial — denial unconsciously deemed necessary for survival as children, and carried on into adulthood. Stage Two Recovery is all about recovering that Inner Child, and bringing him or her to the surface for the world to see and love.

I often use the term *future self* with patients because it is easier for them to conceive of an idealized version of ourselves existing at some point in the future. But by engaging in the process of recovering and asserting our true selves *now*, we quickly move toward an idealized version of ourselves. And as we go about this work, our realities can't help but be favorably impacted.

A by-product of reconnection with our True Self in the present is that we become happier *now*. We don't have to wait around for our circumstances to catch up with the idealized future world in which we aspire to walk. Authenticity makes the journey far more enjoyable.

In quantum terms, regaining and asserting our authenticity *now* enables us to become better tuned-in to the quantum reality in which our idealized self resides. In doing so, we become a more powerful and congruent transmitter into the field as well, which expedites our journey.

IT'S ABOUT TIME!

Mathematically-speaking (and our quantum reality reflects this), there is no reason to become stuck in the false belief that time only functions in one direction. One implication of bi-directional time, of course, is that our present affects our past, as does our future affect *its* past (which includes our present).

So, for us, if an alternative, fully-realized version of ourselves with a strong, coherent electromagnetic signature can affect our current reality — attracting us toward an aspirational ideal — then it's not a stretch to infer that, likewise, a strongly authentic *current* version of ourselves has the potential impact on our past. After all, this week was next week, last week.

ALCHEMY IN REAL LIFE

I had no particular interest in philosophy of mind, time, language, nor physics in the late 80s when I attended undergraduate school at the University of Utah. In fact, I threw a dart at the class bulletin to choose most of my courses, often having procrastinated in their selection to the extent that many of the classes I wanted were already full. At the time, I never imagined, when signing up for them, that I would find them to be intriguing, much less instrumental in my future to the extent that without them this book could not have been written.

The insights gained in those classes have been crucial in my ability to comprehend, and distill, the complex information contained herein, into something understandable to you, the reader. Viewed through the quantum prism, the coincidence of those past choices seems less than coincidental, particularly in light of the more contemporary examples of synchronicities experienced in the process of working on this book.

The quantum worldview provides a powerful clinical tool for decreasing stress in the present by reframing past experiences — some perhaps traumatic — as having been *necessary* to prepare us for our present, or future, circumstances. Granted, we cannot see the future; but, with accurate hindsight we can see how many of our present circumstances are built upon our past. By the same token, there is no reason not to interpret current adversity we may be experiencing as necessary to prepare us for our future.

I've often chuckled at the observation that, "Good judgment comes from experience — which is often the result of bad judgment."

From a practical Stage One Recovery perspective, this interpretation provides *meaning* to our adversity, mitigating its negative emotional impact, and reducing relapse potential. Viktor Frankl was a master at reframing adversity, as exemplified by his masterpiece book, *Man's Search for Meaning*. I highly recommend it.

The idea of viewing past traumas as preparing us for our present or future may seem a bit convenient for some. After all, isn't that a bit like shooting at a tree, and then drawing a bullseye around the bullet hole after the fact? Aren't we making the data fit the conclusion?

One answer is, "Perhaps."

But maybe, at least clinically speaking, the end justifies the means. If, as a clinician, I can help a patient reframe past trauma by changing the *meaning* she assigns to it, thereby mitigating her stress, is that bad?

There may be no concrete proof that every adverse experience we have ever suffered through was meant to serve us; but, what is the harm in *choosing* to view things this way? None. This sort of alchemy turns emotional lead into gold, and at no cost.

Think about it. We have believed a *lot* of things over the years, many of which may or may not have had any basis in reality, but which made us feel like crap. With that in mind, what is the harm in believing something that may or may not have any basis in reality, but which makes us feel *better* about our circumstances?

The problem is that, in the absence of self-awareness, we tend to habitually default to beliefs that cause us distress, as opposed to those that would mitigate it, regardless of their basis in reality. Recognizing this habitual tendency to unconsciously assign negative meanings to our circumstances provides us with a valuable tool to help maintain our emotional center, which is our #1 job in recovery.

You're welcome.

Getting back to my original assertion, you may still ask, "Is bi-directional time real? And is it really possible for our immaterial consciousness to not only have a material impact on the world, but also *retroactively*?"

In the *real* world, in order to avoid making data fit conclusions as we discussed above, scientists have learned to employ clever strategies, such as randomized control groups and double-blind assignment of materials, to ensure no such nonsense ensues.

In *Breaking the Habit of Being Yourself,* Joe Dispenza cites a double-blind study where sepsis patients' health improved faster when they were meditated for by a group of yogis, than did those who were not.

Here is an excerpt from the book:

> In July 2000, Israeli doctor Leonard Leibovici conducted a double-blind, randomized, controlled trial involving 3,393 hospital patients, divided into a control group and an "intercession" group. He set out to see whether prayer could have an effect on their condition. Prayer experiments are great examples of mind affecting matter at a distance. But stay with me here because everything is not always what it seems.

> Leibovici selected patients who had suffered sepsis (an infection) while hospitalized. He randomly designated half the patients to have prayers said for them, while the other half were not prayed for. He compared the results in three categories: how long the fever lasted, length of hospital stays, and how many died as a result of the infection.

> The prayed-for benefited from an earlier decrease in fever and a shorter hospitalization time; the difference in the number of deaths among the prayed-for and not-prayed-for groups was not statistically significant, although better in the prayed-for group. That is a powerful demonstration of the benefits of prayer and

how we can send an intention out into the quantum field through our thoughts and feelings.

However, there's one additional element to this story that you should know about. Did it strike you as slightly odd that in July 2000, a hospital would have more than 3,000 cases of infection at once? Was it a very poorly sterilized place, or was some kind of contagion running rampant? Actually, those who were praying weren't praying for patients who were infected in 2000. Instead, unbeknownst to them, they were praying for lists of people who had been in the hospital from 1990 to 1996 — four to ten years prior to the experiment! The prayed-for patients actually got better during the 1990s from the experiment conducted years later. Let me say this another way: the patients who were prayed for in 2000 all showed measurable changes in health, but those changes took effect years before. A statistical analysis of this experiment proved that these effects were far beyond coincidence. This demonstrates that our intentions, our thoughts and feelings, and our prayers not only affect our present or future, but also, they can actually affect our past as well. Now, this leads to the question: if you were to pray (or focus on an intention) for a better life for yourself, could it affect your past, present, and future? The quantum law says that all potentials exist simultaneously. Our thinking and our feelings affect all aspects of life, beyond both space and time.

The punch line in the study cited above is that the patients, both those being meditated for, and those not meditated for, underwent medical treatment *years prior* to the time the experiment was conducted. Yet the outcomes for those who received meditational prayers were better than for those who did not. So, time, it turns out, is *not* experienced the same way in quantum reality as in our day to day lives.

As I ponder my infatuation with those Philosophy of Time and Philosophy of Mind classes back in undergrad school, I had no idea that the seeds planted then would serve a meaningful purpose in my future. Sure, I was absorbed by the material; but, I *arbitrarily* chose those classes from the semester catalog one day while trying to fill my schedule enough to qualify for student loans. Yet, were it not for that bit of (good?) fortune, this book would never have become a reality.

The Delayed Choice Quantum Eraser experiment, the Fabric of the Mind content in the *Nature of Time* episode, and the mathematics that define quantum mechanics, conspire to force us to conclude that time does, in fact, work both ways.

So, when you have clear aspirations, understand that from a quantum perspective, your ideal future self is reaching across spacetime to guide you toward it.

HOW UNCERTAINTY WORKS

When patients express fear of the unknown citing inability to predict their future, Dispenza likes to say, "The best way to predict your future is to create it from the unknown," and he's right. *Without* change we know what the past brings, and the future will likely continue to bring — finite possibilities. But the uncertainty inherent to quantum mechanics affords us *hope*, and should be embraced rather than feared.

Uncertainty in quantum reality is best illustrated by the famed double-slit experiment that demonstrates not only uncertainty, but also, how we, through application of our immaterial consciousness, affect material change — creating our future *from* uncertainty. The fuzzy nature of the present, or more precisely, *now*, means that past performance does not guarantee future results. In fact, it is a scientifically proven fact that constant change and possibility is the default state of the present in quantum reality — *not* stasis.

As conscious beings, we *partner* with the Universe in designing our life. This is done by aspirationally-driven, guided meditations, as well as by managing our focus as we go throughout our day to day lives.

Review the video below to gain some insight into the double-slit experiment and its implications for how consciousness influences reality — a concept integral to the UTR clinical model.

The way the experiment works is explained in the video. In a nutshell, if we shoot electrons *one at a time* toward a double-slitted barrier between an electron gun particle source and a sensor screen, an "interference pattern" will slowly formulate as the electrons hit the sensor screen one at a time (see left-hand illustration below).

It is as though the electron began as a particle as it left the electron gun, and then as soon as it left the electron gun, turned into a wave (had it not, there would be no interference pattern), and then collapsed back into particle form just in time to transfer its energy onto the sensor screen as a single point or particle once again.

This, in itself, is interesting as we ponder *how* the (material) particle seemingly converts to wave (energy) form, and then back into particle after it travels through the barrier but before hitting the screen. And how does it "know" *where* to (and not to) hit the sensor screen?

Bizarrely, when we *know* (through conscious observation) which path the electron took through the barrier, by placing sensors at the slits, an interference pattern no longer forms on the sensor screen, but rather a "clump" pattern (right-hand illustration above) that corresponds to the straight-line path between the electron gun and the sensor screen. This suggests that *the act of conscious observation of the wave/particle system* actually collapsed the wave into a particle *solely* by virtue of its being observed, resulting in the particle no longer being a wave (along with the wave's inherent uncertainty). Our *knowledge* of the system impacts the outcome. When we do not *know* which slit a particle went through, the system acts as though the particle went through both slits, creating an interference pattern. When we *know* which slit the particle went through, it acts like a particle, creating a clump pattern. In other words, the system clearly *knows* when we are aware of certain aspects of its state. Consciousness materially impacts reality. But are subatomic particles sentient? Do they have awareness? If so, how?

CONSCIOUS OBSERVATION CONVERTS IMMATERIAL POSSIBILITY INTO MATERIAL REALITY

A central mystery

The classic double slit experiment seems to suggest quantum objects such as electrons are sometimes **particles**, sometimes **waves** – and we decide which guise they take

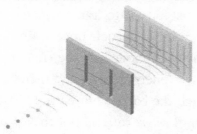 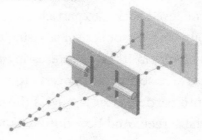

A stream of single electrons is fired at two slits and measured on a screen behind. An interference pattern forms, as if each electron were a **wave** that passed through both slits at once

Measure the electrons first at the slits, however, and you see individual **particles** passing through one slit or the other – and the interference pattern on the screen disappears

Notable is the fact that the act of observation is not *touching* anything. This fact is at odds with Newtonian mechanics, which states that immediate proximity is a necessary condition for change to occur to whatever is being changed. Yet, we have just seen how consciousness, which is immaterial, plays a role in changing the state of the double-slit system. Proximity to the system is irrelevant. In fact, in a later chapter, we will see how people meditating on a similar system are able to impact the outcomes of the experiment from the other side of the planet.

"How does this double-slit stuff relate to recovery?" you might ask. Well, the simple answer goes back to the concept of learned helplessness.

In the classical, macro-, Newtonian world of day to day life we probably have good reason to assume that stasis, or minimal change, is the norm as time progresses along. *An object at rest tends to stay at rest unless acted upon by an outside force* — right? But the nature of quantum mechanics is that reality's default resting state is one of *unrest* or uncertainty. In fact, considering the fuzzy, immaterial energy-state of the unobserved universe, it's miraculous that we are *not* constantly changing from moment to moment.

Richard Feynman's *Infinite Paths* model (which we will cover in the next chapter) explains the relatively stable nature of our current timeline and states that our present reality, or *now*, is completely unpredictable until acted upon by *conscious intention*.

All we need to do is scale up the double-slit experiment, whereby conscious intention, or awareness, converts one electron wave of possibility into a material electron. In doing so, we then affect our macro-reality.

With this understanding, we must necessarily accept the fact that our past performance has *nothing* to do with our

future prospects. We need no longer fear life with a limited future, or what Joe Dispenza would call *a finite signature.*

Life *truly is* mind over matter.

Two additional points explained in the videos on the double-slit experiment with implications for UTR are the following:

1. Richard Feynman's *infinite paths* perspective mentioned briefly in the previous video (and fully explained later) reveals that ALL possible realities simultaneously exist in a state of *superposition.* This, plus the fact that consciousness directs reality, makes it clear that we *select* our reality moment-to-moment from an infinite range of possibilities at any (actually *every*) given point in time.

2. If we want to believe in *object permanence* (that the moon doesn't disappear when we're not looking) *and* that conscious observation is required for conversion from immaterial energy state into material state, then it is logical to infer some sort of Universal Consciousness or Divine Intelligence is *thinking* about the moon, and arguably everything else that no one else is thinking about.

According to Joe Dispenza, "The quantum field is just waiting for a conscious observer to come along and influence energy in the form of potential matter by using the mind and consciousness to make waves of potential energetic probabilities coalesce into physical matter." He gets it. On the upside, managing our focus is a great tool for emotional self-regulation and is critical to our recovery process as well as relapse prevention. How we direct our consciousness also influences our reality. Everything we have ever accomplished was, at one point, just a thought. Once we really internalize the nature of reality, particularly the direct relationship between mind and matter, the importance of managing our focus becomes quite obvious.

In the absence of self-awareness, particularly in light of the habitual negative outlook addiction imposes on us over time, we are likely to negatively impact our reality in very concrete ways. Suddenly, resolving unconscious thinking errors (see Chapter 5) becomes more than just a rhetorical exercise. It becomes critical to our happiness, and our ability to design an ideal world for ourselves.

PROOF THAT MIND OVER MATTER WORKS

The following lecture by Dean Radin cites a number of scientific studies including his own, all of which prove that consciousness in fact impacts material reality. A stronger statement would be that our reality is material evidence of the application of consciousness. Of note in his findings is the fact that proximity to that which is being influenced is irrelevant — more evidence of "spooky action at a distance", disconfirming conventional wisdom.

So again we see that consciousness (energy), and the material world are inextricably connected — the quantum field being the common denominator in both. We'll flesh that out later, but the irrefutable fact that consciousness affects reality makes us, in a manner of speaking, supernatural. We create, or select, our reality by focusing our intention.

We are literally the authors of our destiny.

The image below is a two-dimensional rendering of what would be a helium atom's three-dimensional "probability cloud." Each pinpoint dot represents the probable location of its electron, if measured. Until it is consciously measured for position, the electron does not materialize. The darker the shade, the greater the probability of its appearance in that specific location. BUT unless measured, the electron is in wave, or immaterial form. Its possible trajectory can be measured, but not its position. The moment its position is attempted to be measured by a conscious observer, it is no longer in wave form — this phenomenon is known as "collapsing the wave function." The dots in the illustration do not represent actual locations. Each point represents a *possible* location. This is the fuzzy nature of reality, which remains completely uncertain until coalesced into reality by a conscious observer.

In the UTR clinical model, we simply scale up this single subatomic particle concept to the macro level of everyday existence, leveraging the fuzzy nature of reality to create change *in the now*, both in ourselves and in the reality in which we walk.

PROBABILITY CLOUD — FUZZY REALITY

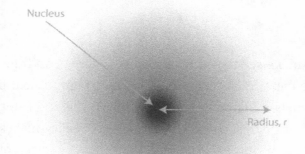

Nucleus

Radius, r

In the next video, Arvin Ash illustrates how the uncertainty conceptualized by the Heisenberg Uncertainty Principle plays out in our macro world:

 12.10

The Heisenberg Uncertainty Principle implies that the nature of the world is not deterministic, continuous, nor logical by any conventional standard.

One takeaway for me from this video is the mathematics Dr. Ash cites that enable precise predictions. The nature and role of mathematics will become crucial later as we ponder the essence, function, and origin of the quantum fields.

The following, easily digestible video accomplishes two things relating to recovery quite well.

A. It explains how the implications of the Heisenberg Uncertainty Principle provide a basis for belief in our ability to affect *immediate* change in our life.

B. It illustrates how Quantum Entanglement provides a proven scientific basis for connection between current, past, and future aspirational versions of ourselves across time and timelines.

▷ 12.11

Quantum entanglement lends plausibility to UTR's assertion that our past and present aspirations reflect the existence of a mutually-entangled version of our most realized self in the quantum field of possibilities, to which we, with our unique electromagnetic signature, are attuned.

In light of this assertion, a fair question to bring up would be, "How would proponents of UTR account for people's shifting aspirations over time?" For example, at different times in their life, a person may have wanted to be a pilot, a lawyer, a rock star, an electrician, and a chemist. Isn't this problematic? In a word, no. In fact, there are many plausible responses to this question:

1. With an infinite number of potential realities available, fully-realized versions of *all* possible outcomes exist. It is that to which our current self is most attuned that inspires us aspirationally toward it.

2. Many aspirations, particularly prior to an individual's reconnecting with their True Self, are false, particularly if adopted to align with another's agenda out of fear of abandonment.

3. We can always organically change our minds as we evolve. With infinite possibilities, we're not going to run out of more-realized versions of ourselves — ever.

4. We may achieve one aspirational reality, get bored, and then move on to another.

5. We may move in and out of Authenticity as environmental factors interfere.

6. We may reach an aspirational state, realize we were thinking too small, and re-engage the Universe toward another ideal reality.

SUMMARY

STAGE 1 RECOVERY — PREVENT RELAPSE

+ Understanding the true nature of the Universe helps us to understand how we influence our reality, which creates hope and reduces anxiety — making us creators rather than victims.

+ When we realize that we can leverage the quantum nature of the Universe to affect our reality, with little effort, anxiety is decreased, hope is increased, and thus relapse potential is diminished.

+ Understanding that the present affects the past helps accept current adversity as necessary and survivable. This knowledge decreases stress by giving adversity meaning beyond immediate suffering.

STAGE 2 RECOVERY — REGAIN AUTHENTICITY

+ Understanding who we are, and the role we play in creating our reality encourages us to recover our True Selves.

+ When we see the realities we have experienced in an inauthentic state, and the unhappiness that ensued, we can see the value in reconnecting with our True Self and manifesting a reality based upon that which we truly want in life as opposed to realizing others' agenda for us.

STAGE 3 RECOVERY — ENHANCE SPIRITUAL CAPACITY

+ We and the Universe are co-authors of our reality.

+ Realizing our capacity to influence our reality by leveraging the Universe to our own end.

+ Feedback provided by the Universe in our authentic state of being, reinforces our decision to recover our True Selves, and creates excitement at possibility, defeating learned helplessness.

+ Making sense of our past, and the fact that we have not only survived adversity, but also, learned and thrived from it, helps us to realize that past suffering has prepared us to become the person we are now — capable of enlightenment — and on the path toward realizing a potential only dreamed of before gaining this insight.

CHAPTER 13

HOW QUANTUM FIELDS WORK

REDUCTIONISM VS. HOLISM

Are we — our True Self — matter or energy? And what might the implications be to the answer to this question? We will find out later that the question itself is faulty. In formal logic terms, it is fallacious in that it presumes there are only two choices — the *False Choice Fallacy*. However, it was not considered fallacious as recently as the turn of the twenty-first century due to the limitations of our scientific knowledge at the time.

This is important because it illustrates the principle that often our *questions* are limited by our current understanding. When the questions at hand are supposed to lead us to enlightenment about how reality works, gaps in our knowledge can become problematic because they serve as pretext for our questions. Until field theory was developed and then proven, either-or questions, such as "are we material or energy", led to a dead end.

Exploring the edge of our understanding where philosophy and science intersect is where all the fun is. We learn the most when we ask questions that seemingly have no answers. By spending time there, we learn about both ourselves *and* reality.

Necessity truly is the mother of invention.

My favorite class back in undergrad was "Philosophy of Mind", which used a textbook entitled, *The Mind's I*. I still have the original paperback used for that class, which is now tattered and in awful shape, having been referred to so many times over the decades since, for recreational reading. An excerpt from the book's introduction is as follows:

> *You see the moon rise in the east. You see the moon rise in the west. You watch two moons moving toward each other across the cold black sky, one soon to pass behind the other as they continue on their way. You are on Mars, millions of miles from home, protected from the killing frostless cold of the red Martian desert by fragile membranes of terrestrial technology. Protected but stranded; for your spaceship has broken down beyond repair. You will never again return to Earth, to the friends and family and places you left behind.*
>
> *But perhaps there is hope. In the communication compartment of the disabled craft you find a Teleclone Mark IV teleporter and instructions for its use. If you turn the teleporter on, tune its beam to the Telecone receiver on Earth, and then step into the sending chamber, the teleporter will swiftly and painlessly dismantle your body, producing a molecule-by-molecule blueprint, which will be beamed to Earth, where the receiver, its reservoirs well stocked with the requisite atoms, will almost instantaneously produce, from the beamed instructions — you! Whisked back to Earth at the speed of light, into the arms of your loved ones, who*

will soon be listening with rapt attention to your tales of adventures on Mars.

One last survey of the damaged spaceship convinces you that the Teleclone is your only hope. With nothing to lose, you set the transmitter up, flip the right switches, and step into the chamber — 5 4, 3, 2, 1, FLASH! You open the door in front of you and step out of the Teleclone receiver chamber into the sunny, familiar atmosphere of Earth. You've come home, none the worse for wear after your long-distance Teleclone fall from Mars. Your narrow escape from a terrible fate on the red planet calls for a celebration; and, as your family and friends gather around, you notice how everyone as changed since you last saw them. It has been almost three years, after all, and you've all grown older. Look at Sarah, your daughter, who must now be eight and a half. You find yourself thinking "Can this be the little girl who used to sit on my lap?" Of course it is, you reflect, even though you must admit that you do not so much recognize her as extrapolate from memory and deduce her identity. She is so much taller, looks so much older, and knows so much more. In fact, most of the cells in her body were not there when you last cast eyes on her. But in spite of growth and change, in spite of replacement cells, she's still the same little person you kissed goodbye three years ago.

Then it hits you: "Am I, really, the same person who kissed this little girl goodbye three years ago? Am I this eight-year-old child's mother or am I, actually, a brand-new human being, only several hours old, in spite of my memories — or apparent memories — of days and years before that? Did this child's mother recently die on Mars, dismantled, and destroyed in the chamber of a Teleclone Mark IV?

The cutting-edge argument in the scientific and philosophical world at the time *The Mind's I* was published was the so-called mind-body problem that involved two camps: Cartesian and Reductionist. The above passage reflects the concept of quantum entanglement illustrated in the Fabric of the Cosmos series in which they discussed teleportation.

The Cartesian camp simply asserts that consciousness is distinct and separate from our material existence. This is the *ghost in the machine* argument, if you will, that presumes a clear distinction between *brain* and *mind*. A spiritual essence is inferred in the Cartesian model — named after the French philosopher Descartes whose worldview was more aligned with the religious paradigm prevalent at the time — souls, consciousness, etc. — than it was with his scientific contemporaries.

The Reductionist perspective states that brains are no more than a collection of atoms, and it is by virtue of their architecture they create what we perceive as consciousness. This worldview requires no higher power.

The Reductionist approach never intuitively resonated with me; but, at the time I was unwilling to take the leap of faith necessary to adopt a spiritual perspective, having no particularly compelling reason to do so. Plus, I was attending The University of Utah, which was situated in a predominantly religious state, and being a contrarian was far more interesting than surrendering my will (and 10 percent of my income) to the General Authority representing the local religion at the time.

At the time *The Mind's I* was written in the 80s, particle theory was the frontier of our understanding of the nature of the Universe. The best argument, at that time in favor of a higher power, was simply to assert one — consciousness itself being *circumstantial evidence* thereof. This circular argument was understandably rejected by purist physicists who believed there was still lots of 'splainin' to do.

Thirty years later, it turns out that *both* models — Reductionist and Cartesian — are accurate, because as we will soon discover, nothing *is* something.

Quantum Field Theory was first proposed as a mathematical theory. It was eventually proven experimentally, over time, as scientific instruments capable of testing it became available. Fermi-Lab and The Large Hadron Collider near Geneva, Switzerland, were instrumental in filling out the picture, gradually reconciling particle and quantum mechanics, and ultimately, enabling consciousness to be seriously considered for integration into our understanding of reality.

In this section I have three video links — all selected for their unique contribution to understanding fields, which are the fundamental building blocks from which everything in the universe is *derived*. Seventeen fields have been identified, although everything in our observable world is derived from just a handful of them. The final field, the key to conversion from energy to material state — the Higgs boson field — was scientifically substantiated in 2012 by the LHC, built by CERN in Switzerland.

One of the most substantial yet understandable and entertaining lectures on the nature of fields is presented in the following video, by David Tong:

 13.1

The illustration below identifies the 17 fields. If they did not work in *perfect* concert, reality as we know it would not exist. Period.

The little number in the upper left-hand corner of each box is of particular interest. This number represents the exact amount of energy necessary to generate exactly one subatomic particle from that field. For example, that value in the upper-left-hand *up quark* box is 2.2MeV/c2 or 2.2 mega-electron volts per square centimeter.

Perturbations, or small electromagnetic disturbances within the fields, are what generate each of the subatomic particles that make up you and me. These perturbations *must* contain no more or less than each box's value in order to convert energy into mass (a particle).

Standard Model of Elementary Particles

This concept shook the foundation of my understanding of whom (or *what*) I am. We are literally 100 percent *derivative* of these fields. Virtual holograms. Our bodies' smallest components — subatomic particles, are *fleeting* in nature. Nearly *virtual*. (I hope there aren't any power outages in the quantum field any time soon!)

Everything we call real is made up
of things we can't call real.

— Niels Bohr

I ran across a social media post in my feed from a year ago during the beginning of my research for this book, which was just an idea at the time. The post reads, *"We study subatomic particles because we hope to learn about ourselves — after all, we're made of them."* This startled me a bit because when I think of the term, *myself*, I don't really visualize myself as being a bunch of subatomic particles. Studying subatomic particles is not learning about *myself* — it's learning about subatomic particles. Or is it?

When I was introduced to Quantum Field Theory I realized that quantum fields provide the scientifically-proven construct for unifying consciousness, spirituality, and our physical being because *consciousness and the quantum fields are energy.*

To put it another way: **We are far more ghost than machine.**

The fields provide continuous connection between literally everyone and everything in the universe.

There are 12 Scalar and 5 Vector fields, all massless and immaterial, which serve as the source of every single subatomic particle (mass) comprising every single thing in the universe — you, me, your chair, the floor under your chair, air, the building you are in, the earth, moon, planets, sun, stars, your beverage — literally everything in the universe. Everything you see is 100 percent derivative of precise energy "perturbations" in the fields yielding their associated subatomic particles. Three quark and one electron field produce everything in the visible world. The other fields' associated subatomic particles serve no day-to-day practical purpose we can discern at this time.

I like this next video because of the clarity with which Arvin Ash breaks down these concepts, and for the visualizations he uses to illustrate them. Something that really sticks out to me in his presentation is the seemingly transient nature of the subatomic particles that make us up. This supports the notion that we not only *can* change in short order, but also, a state of constant flux is at the heart of our very nature.

The presentation does a great job explaining the mechanism by which the subatomic particles that comprise everything in the universe come into being — disappearing and reappearing as fields' energy concentrations fluctuate in a seemingly random manner. In one of his YouTube videos, Joe Dispenza asserts that we fluctuate in and out of the fields 7.8 times per second.

The following presentation is the best rendering I have found showing how all of the fields work in unison.

The video illustrates the intricate dynamics at play in the behavior of two subatomic particles. Imagine the number of things that have to go *right* to produce the complex reality we know.

HOW SCALAR FIELDS WORK

Fields come in two types — scalar (of which there are 12) and vector (there are 5 of these). In a nutshell, scalar fields *yield or generate* particles, and vector fields *govern the behavior* of said particles.

The subatomic particles that comprise the atoms, which is everything that you and I observe in our three-dimensional world, are primarily derived from three scalar fields. Those scalar fields produce atoms' component up-quarks, down-quarks (comprising atomic nuclei) and electrons (which are free-standing particles not necessarily tethered to an atom).

The mechanism by which a particle comes into existence — from a field state of pure *energy* into a *material* state — begins as a *perturbation*, which takes place when a scalar field is excited to a very specific energy level. If you consult the previous diagram, you can see the amount of energy required to produce each type of particle noted in the upper left-hand corner of each box corresponding to its fundamental particle.

For instance, in order to bring an *up quark* (1/3 of a proton) into material existence from its potential or immaterial state, an electrical charge exactly equal to 2.2 mega-electron volts per centimeter squared of energy is required in its field. Any less, and the *up quark* field will not bring any particle into existence. Exactly 2x that charge will produce exactly two *up quarks*, and so on. The nucleus of an atom consists of protons and neutrons. A proton consists of two *up quarks* and one *down quark*, and a neutron consists of two *down quarks* and one *up quark*. One proton and one neutron comprise a helium atom's nucleus, and its (the helium atom's) one electron requires .511 mega-electron volts per centimeter squared of energy to be brought into existence from its unique field.

The Higgs Field is special because it enables the perturbations in the scalar fields to turn energy into mass (particles). Without the Higgs Field, nothing would form nor exist in the universe.

Discovery of the Higgs boson field by the Large Hadron Collider near Geneva, Switzerland, in 2012, constituted proof of the missing field, completing what is now referred to as *The Standard Model* of the universe (see diagram below), which accurately predicts the result of *every single experiment ever done in science*. It shows us how reality works.

THE STANDARD MODEL

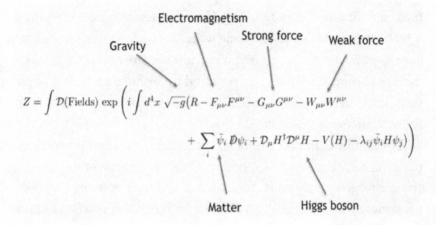

HOW VECTOR FIELDS WORK

The Gluon field, referred to in the above diagram as Strong Force, is the vector field responsible for the so-called conservation of angular momentum *within* atoms' nucleus, keeping its component subatomic particles from flying off willy-nilly. The Gluon field keeps the atoms' protons and neutron quarks stuck together to form the nucleus of atoms. Think, *gluon = glue*.

The W and Z Boson Fields, represented by the Weak Force reference in the above equation, keep atoms' electrons from flying off until they interact with another atom's electrons. They also account for, among other things, radioactivity. But that is irrelevant for our purposes, as are other vector fields' specific functions at this time; but, suffice it to know that they all play roles in how reality works.

Conceptually speaking, vector fields govern the behavior of the scalar fields' derivative particles. In other words vector fields contain the *rules*, or *laws* by which material reality and the universe are defined.

In the videos thus far, you have seen numerous instances where mathematics is applied to explain relationships and abstractions. These maths are *baked into* both the vector and scalar fields accounting for our ability to explain, predict, or extrapolate anything we encounter in the universe with supreme precision.

Some of the more familiar mathematical abstractions that manifest as properties of the vector fields include:

CONSERVATION OF ANGULAR MOMENTUM

The angular momentum of an isolated system remains constant in both magnitude and direction. The angular momentum is defined as the product of the moment of inertia I and the angular velocity. The angular momentum is a vector quantity, and the vector sum of the angular momenta of the parts of an isolated system is constant. As far as we can tell, conservation of angular momentum is an absolute symmetry of nature. That is, we do not know of anything in nature that violates it.

CONSERVATION OF MOMENTUM

The momentum of an isolated system is a constant. The vector sum of the momenta mv of all the objects of a system cannot be changed by interactions within the system. This puts a strong constraint on the types of motions that can occur in an isolated system. If one part of the system is given a momentum in a given direction, then some other part or parts of the system must simultaneously be given exactly the same momentum in the opposite direction. As far as we can tell, conservation of momentum is an absolute symmetry of nature. That is, we do not know of anything in nature that violates it.

CONSERVATION OF ENERGY

Energy can be defined as the capacity for doing work. It may exist in a variety of forms and may be transformed from one type of energy to another. However, these energy transformations are constrained by a fundamental principle, the Conservation of Energy principle. One way to state this principle is "Energy can neither be created nor destroyed." Another approach is to say that the total energy of an isolated system remains constant.

Without these laws, or mathematical abstractions, the universe as we know it would not exist. These laws all apply to *closed systems*, which implies that the universe is a closed system. This will become relevant when we drill through field theory to the core of reality — information.

So, as you can see, each field is highly specialized, and were any of them defective, nothing we would recognize would be in the universe, which would be a moot point because we would not be here (exist) to recognize anything either.

The final field discovered went from theory to scientifically accepted reality in 2012. The importance of this field cannot be overstated because it gives subatomic particles their mass (enabling their conversion from immaterial energy to material mass). This is the Higgs boson field. The best video I have encountered explaining this thus far is the following:

13.4

Grasping these concepts can be a challenge, but none of them need to be fully understood for us to derive the necessary value to move forward. Just absorb what you can, internalize it with practice, and then go back for more. The more I understand these principles, the more conviction I have in them, and in our ability to leverage them to our benefit.

Periodic Table of the Elements

Every element in the universe (see above) is derivative of the fields' perfect interaction. Field-directed forces enable the chemical interactions that yield everything — even us (our bodies).

The following is a comprehensive paper by Timo Weigand at Heidelberg University into the nature of quantum field theory. The amount of mathematics will prove salient as we approach the edge of our understanding:

13.5

The takeaway thus far is that fields are real, immaterial and indivisible, and constitute the very fabric of reality — and most importantly serve as the mechanism by which consciousness and pure energy is converted to material reality.

Let us summarize for a moment the nature of reality in Field terms:

- The universe's fundamental building blocks are the 17 fields (energy).
- At any given point in time superposition of infinite *potential* realities may be collapsed into *material* reality by conscious observation (intention).
- The quantum field and consciousness are inextricable from each other.
- Quantum mechanics and the field enable us to influence material reality.
- Without fields there would *literally* be nothing, not even consciousness.
- As energy in the form of a consciousness, and inextricable from the quantum field, we are all connected to each other and the Universe.
- The field is the vehicle by which we as conscious beings with dual citizenship commune with a higher power or divine consciousness that is infused throughout the field.

EVERYTHING ALL THE TIME

Richard Feynman's *Infinite Quantum Paths* model, which is central to the UTR clinical model, is based on the quantum mechanics relating consciousness and matter (collapse of the wave function). However, rather than collapsing an individual wave function into a single particle, the principle is simply scaled up.

The following video explains the simultaneous superposition of all possible worlds — infinite possibility — now. One conclusion arrived at in Feynman's work is that *everything not observed that can happen, does happen.*

 13.6

The presenter in the Feynman video also says that the Universe is *lazy*. This is a reference to the Principle of Least Action, which is basically a quantum take on the Newtonian law of inertia that (you may recall from high school physics class) states that "an object at rest tends to remain at rest unless acted upon by an outside force." In the quantum realm this means that, absent conscious engagement, or strong congruent *intention* in the field, our trajectory or life path will remain fairly predictable. In UTR, the outside force responsible for changing our reality is our consciousness, amplified by emotion, in a meditative state.

Those not exposed to UTR concepts tend to either believe that they cannot change, or that even if they do manage, there is a fairly narrow range of possibilities — none sufficiently compelling to justify a solid effort — so they don't try. This type of stagnant thinking is simply inaccurate and must be overcome in recovery if we are to affect profound change.

Mathematically speaking, another way to think about this concept of the Universe being lazy is the philosophical concept of Occam's Razor, which states that, given a number of options, the simplest explanation is usually the correct one. Webster's Dictionary puts it more concisely:

*(Occam's razor is) a scientific and philosophical rule that enti-
ties should not be multiplied unnecessarily, which is interpreted
as requiring that the simplest of competing theories be preferred
over the more complex, or that explanations of unknown phe-
nomena be sought first in terms of known quantities.*

Logically-speaking, a given life-path, or reality (of the infinite
number always available) will experience little change without some
conscious effort. In UTR, that effort comes in the form of a medi-
tated-upon clear, idealized vision for ourselves and corresponding
ideal reality, leveraging quantum mechanics as opposed to laboring
along in a Newtonian manner with little substantial impact.

The superposition of every possible reality at every single point
in time affords us the means to dramatically affect our reality. In
essence, we can select moment to moment from an infinite number of possible timelines — one of which will materialize with the
application of our conscious intentions in a meditative state.

The UTR clinical model is *not* a classical linear cause-and-effect, effort-based Newtonian model like most change models. With
UTR, creating change is more like switching the stations on a TV
with infinite channels, each corresponding to a possible future or
timeline. Each "channel" is a lifepath — one of which contains our
idealized self and reality. Incremental lateral moves are set into
motion by conscious intentionality, requiring *much* less effort than
traditional change because the Universe does all of the heavy lifting.

From a recovery perspective this enables us to employ the Universe to our advantage rather than feel like *we* have to affect every
single outcome ourselves. By integrating this concept into our worldview, we become less overwhelmed because we realize that we
need not produce *every* desired outcome through our individual,

physical effort. This realization fosters hope and decreases stress, both of which are clinically beneficial.

SUMMARY

STAGE 1 RECOVERY — PREVENT RELAPSE

+ Realizing we are not who we thought we were creates an exciting new self-concept without limitations.
+ The possibility of change, and a stronger identification with the Universe, decreases stress. Hopelessness and stress are replaced with curiosity, wonder, and hope about the future.
+ A compelling future vision minimizes the perceived necessity for drugs and alcohol, and cravings.

STAGE 2 RECOVERY — REGAIN AUTHENTICITY

+ When we realize that there is no possible reality that does not exist, and that recovering our True Self affords us the best possibility of moving toward a fully realized reality in which gratitude is our default state, we become committed to asserting our True Self now, making us happier in the process.
+ When we understand how quantum entanglement works with our True Self, our resolve for authenticity outweighs fear of being judged by others.
+ In our new state of authenticity, some may revolve out of our lives, but the *right* people will revolve into it — people who love us for who we are, and for no other reason.

STAGE 3 RECOVERY — ENHANCE SPIRITUAL CAPACITY

+ As we gain experience in asserting our True Selves, and experience feedback from the Universe aligned with our aspirations, we gain momentum toward faith.

+ Understanding Feynman's Infinite Paths (multiverse) theory opens us to the possibility that we need not unnecessarily exert ourselves to affect outcomes. We simply need clarity of vision afforded us by our True Self. This realization not only defeats learned helplessness, but perpetuates our capacity to adopt a spiritual perspective.

CHAPTER 14

HOW ASPIRATION WORKS

Quantum entanglement is one of the most important aspects to grasp if we are to understand the connection between our current and idealized selves.

The principles outlined in the video below are relevant to UTR for a number of reasons. Quantum entanglement is one of many concepts we apply after analyzing the results of the *Magic Wand Thought Experiment* fleshed out earlier in the book. Combined with the bi-directionality of time, and Feynman's Infinite Paths theory, entanglement provides the mechanism whereby our aspirations may be interpreted as *future memories* of an already-existing idealized version of ourselves. That fully-realized self and corresponding reality serve as a beacon on the horizon for us, providing motivation, clarity, hope, and guidance in selecting the values we need to move in that direction. In the present, if done properly, that idealized vision becomes infinitely more compelling than, say, substance use.

▷ 14.1

In scientific terms, Joe Dispenza would say that the fully-realized version of ourselves has a strong, coherent electromagnetic signature to which we are attuned — that our present and fully-realized versions of ourselves are quantum-entangled in the manner described in the video.

Joseph Campbell would add that the idealized version we have envisioned resonates with our *current* Authentic Self, prompting the Universe to respond to our aspirational pursuits.

According to ACA's account of Stage Three Recovery, it is *only* through the True Self that we most effectively connect with a higher power.

Quantum entanglement, as outlined in the companion videos, is a common element of *all* of these independently developed paradigms: ACA, anthropological mythology, Eastern spiritual philosophy, and now, UTR.

Bonus: Reconnecting with our Authentic Self not only facilitates movement toward our ideal self and enables connection to a higher power, but authenticity helps resolve low self-esteem in the present. As such, we become happier *now* as we work toward self-realization.

"KNOWERS"

Earlier on, I alluded to the preponderance of mathematics encountered when physicists explain the nature of reality. An example of this is provided in the following video:

▶ 14.2

Although the content in the above video is interesting, what is more interesting for our purposes is that, in it, Arvin Ash indirectly alludes to the existence of a divine *knower* when he attempts to explain why the macro-world does not *appear* to act the same way as the micro-world. He uses terms like, ". . . there must be no record made anywhere in the Universe . . ." or ". . . the Universe could examine all the photons in the box . . .", which implies that the Universe either has or is a consciousness able to observe the "data" or information put out by the subatomic particles contained in the box. In the quantum realm, observation is a key aspect to defining reality — presumably in his example, observation by the Universe Itself.

David Tong, in his lecture on quantum fields, asserted that the fields preceded the Big Bang, or were at the very least, present at the exact moment of the beginning of the Universe, resulting in the irregularities responsible for uneven distribution of matter, which in turn enabled the formation of stars, galaxies, and everything material.

Although there is intelligence and precision built into the fields, rather than attribute this to a divine source, Tong simply states, "We don't know why this is the way it is." — which is fine for him.

In fact, Arvin Ash, as well as *all* of the physicists encountered throughout the course of my research for this book, adamantly reject the idea of either deferring to, or inferring a higher power to fill the gaps in their knowledge.

People have been presuming all-powerful gods to explain things they did not yet understand since the dawn of humanity. When the weather turned bad, for instance, ancient humans concluded that *the gods must be angry.* Had everyone simply accepted these explanations for how the world works, we would have ceased making the very discoveries that have led to the depth of understanding we now hold as to the nature of reality and the universe.

Physics visionaries such as Copernicus, DaVinci, and Galileo took their very lives in their hands by espousing findings that ran counter to the conventional wisdom of the day, or dogma, held by the powers that be.

Talk about Cancel Culture!!

Although the fields are the nervous system connecting everything in the universe — instantly — information is the basis of everything including the fields themselves, and must have come from somewhere. Throughout the supporting video content there are references to "knowers," or to the Universe as an "observer" — the implication being that the Universe either is, or has consciousness. Non-things don't *have* things — like consciousnesses.

Physicists will continue their quest for knowledge. A unified theory of reality — perhaps absent spirituality — may be close at hand, and if accomplished, I don't see how grasping the nature of reality is going to exclude, at least, a *voluntary* spiritual perspective. Thus far, however, the more we learn about the true nature of reality, the more compelling the argument *in favor* of a higher power becomes.

Consider David Tong's aforementioned claim that irregularities in Cosmic Microwave Background Radiation (see illustration below) were caused by quantum field vacuum fluctuations *at the moment* the Big Bang occurred. Were it not for these irregularities, he asserts, galaxies would never have formed — neither would we — due to the absolute uniformity of the initial blast.

COSMIC MICROWAVE BACKGROUND RADIATION

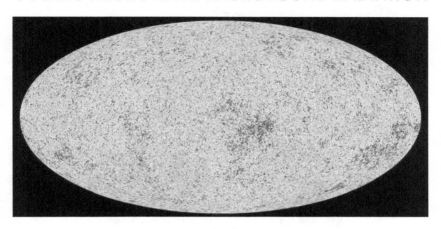

Although the irregularities are interesting in themselves, the *timing* aspect begs the question as to how the fields, which contain such divine algorithms, came into being — and *before* time and the Universe existed?

MATH — PROJECTION OR DISCOVERY?

There is a LOT of math going on in these supporting videos. As my eyes were glazing over with all of the mathematical symbols floating around the screen during one of the videos, a lightbulb went on. I asked myself, "Is math our human way of making sense of the world? Or is math *intrinsic* to the universe?"

In short, is math a matter of projection — or discovery?

I came to the conclusion that since we, and everything in the universe, are all part of the same system — derivative of the quantum fields — then measure*d* and measure*r* are one and the same.

The elegant mathematical axioms defining the vector fields' governance of the motion of subatomic particles, hold true regardless of whether or not they are being measured — so they must be *baked in*to reality. Information, regardless of subjective or objective, has to have *originated somewhere.*

You may recall the segment in *Finding Joe* pointing out that the Chinese symbol for Crisis consists of two characters: the first is *danger*, immediately followed by *opportunity*.

Crisis

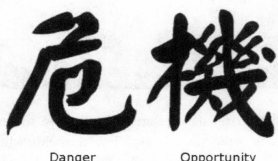

Danger   Opportunity

Before applying this concept to the point at hand, it's worth a few words on its application to Stage One and Two Recovery, particularly for reducing stress.

In dealing with patients who suffer from anxiety, I like to walk them through every crises they have ever experienced. Since I am having this conversation with them, it is fair to presume that they did not die from these crises, even though at the time they may have thought they might.

Without exception, when asked about how they weathered the period after their crises, a theme arises. They invariably learned something about themselves, or others — a lesson they needed to learn. Perhaps the crisis revealed strength they never imagined they had. Perhaps the pain of the event nearly killed them; but, that is exactly what was required in order to get them to realize that the status quo was no longer sustainable. Perhaps their pain forced them to become students of their demise, and in the process, they became so well-versed, they wrote a book with the intention that no one would ever experience the kind of pain they had endured (okay, maybe that's just a hypothetical).

I view crises like airline crashes.

When a plane crashes, they don't race up to it, put the fire out, and then drive off, congratulating themselves on a job well done. No. The National Transportation Safety Board (NTSB) comes out to the scene, they dig up the black boxes — the flight data recorder and cockpit voice recorder — that are usually located in the tail section of all aircraft (which is why I like to sit in the back of the plane — at least they might find me, right?)

The NTSB takes the black boxes, analyzes what happened to cause the crash, and then applies the lessons across the entire industry so that whatever caused the crash *never happens again*. By the same token, we apply the lessons learned from the crises in our lives to prepare us for our futures.

Sadly, those in addiction have diluted access to their emotions; so their crises are usually quite dramatic by most standards.

When we enter recovery and our lives start improving — if we are honest with ourselves — we have no choice but to admit that we *had* to experience every crisis we did, or we would have never gotten the leverage on ourselves to change.

It could have been no other way.

> *Had I not undergone the painful crises I endured as a result of my addictions, I would never have become the person I am proud to say I am today.*

Accepting these facts early in recovery enables us to mitigate feelings of regret, guilt, and shame that would otherwise serve as fuel for potential relapse. Of course, others who may feel victimized by the crises we created may not feel so charitable in their interpretation; but, we can't afford to take responsibility for managing their emotional states, nor is it our responsibility. If they can't see things that way, then so be it. They can choose whether or not they wish to remain in a relationship with us. We have no control over that (see Chapter 5).

Now, back to the point at hand as to how the Chinese character for Crisis applies to the dilemma presented by the mathematics sewn into the fabric of reality.

On the *dilemma or danger* side of the equation is the question: "Where did the exquisite math enabling us and the universe come from?" It's existence implies divine intelligence, but only with circumstantial and circular evidence — the danger being that we can draw no *definitive* conclusion.

On the *opportunity* side of the equation is the question: "Where did the exquisite math enabling us and the universe come from?" — with quantum field theory affording us the most plausible opportunity to date for the introduction of a higher power to our worldview.

Asserting a higher power at this point may feel rather like arranging the data to fit the conclusion. I would rebut that we are connecting the dots between what we *know* to be true scientifically and what we *believe* to be true, *extrapolated* from a mountain of circumstantial evidence.

The more we learn about the nature of reality, the more physics brings us *closer* to spirituality.

ORDER AMONG CHAOS

There is a commonly accepted natural law called *entropy* (the Second Law of Thermodynamics) to which philosophers and cosmologists have subscribed for centuries. This is the Newtonian-era principle behind unidirectional time, which we debunked in a previous chapter.

In day to day life, if we drop a wine glass onto the floor, it breaks into a thousand shards of glass. In *The Fabric of the Cosmos*, David Greene points out that although it is unlikely for us to experience the opposite — shards of glass collecting themselves up into a complete wine glass — within the quantum realm this is not impossible, just implausible. He also points out that getting 1,000 consecutive, *heads,* coin-toss outcomes is also unlikely, although mathematically possible. However, ***in an infinite number of tries, both — in fact, all — scenarios are inevitable.***

The principle of *entropy* asserts that the universe always moves from a state of organization — the ultimate state of organization being the exact moment of the Big Bang — to a state of chaos, or disorganization.

That said, vector fields define with great specificity the behavior of subatomic particles derivative of the scalar fields, enabling them to interact with each other to form atoms and molecules, coalescing into *things* such as you and me, galaxies, paper towel holders, etc. The vector fields contain, and implement, the mathematical laws that govern organization from what *would* be chaos into order.

These laws are in effect at the subatomic level, and thus dictate activity at the macro level.

SOURCE CODE'S SOURCE

The following video by Dr. Jim Al-Khalili left me questioning whether the fields are really the most fundamental component from which the universe is composed. The content of his *Story of*

Information is the ribbon with which I will tie together *all* of the previously covered material.

 14.3

Architecturally-speaking, the fields are fundamental because they are not an abstraction. But information, the theoretical and actual basis for the seventeen quantum fields, *is* an abstraction. It *means stuff.*

Given *Information Theory* presented in the documentary, and our understanding of quantum mechanics as a backdrop, one must then ask:

- Does information *mean* anything if there's no one there to perceive it?
- Is information *intended* to mean anything?
  If so, by "whom"?
- Does information require consciousness to be meaningful?
- Does information exist in the absence of consciousness?
- Is all information everywhere all the time?
- Does information travel faster than light?
- Does the same information mean different things to different entities?
- Where does information come from?
- Does information ever go anywhere?
- What is the relationship between the fields and information?
- Is information energy?
- Is all of the information here in the universe?
  - If so, what are the implications?

The answers to some of these questions can be resolved by introducing a higher power. I suspect that science will provide definitive answers to these questions in the future.

But before getting ahead of ourselves, let us explore the nature of information in greater depth.

Information is the basis for *everything*. The truth is that nothing is independent of information.

As noted in many of the prior videos, the universe is a closed system. That means that ALL of the information in the universe is already there. That said, it must have come from *somewhere* — it could not *not* have.

Information is encoded into the fields. And the fields function in a *perfect*, mathematically-prescribed manner. Yet it is important to note that information always requires a medium (such as a consciousness).

The scalar fields constantly produce subatomic particles, which the vector fields then manipulate. These subatomic particles are coalesced into atoms, those atoms into molecules, and then into rocks, or trees, organic tissues, and even into people who read books on spirituality. We are information in physiological form. We go about our daily lives as information coded into our trillions of DNA strands derivative, ultimately, of the quantum field.

Everything is the way it is because of how information defines it. And information is the way it is because of what?

HOW WE ARE LIKE HOLOGRAMS

Toward the end of the *Fabric of the Cosmos* NOVA series episode on Space, a theory was put forth. Discussing the nature of black holes, the episode pointed out that when anything is sucked into one, despite its three-dimensional properties no longer being intact, *all* of the information contained within it remains. This theory coincides with the video on information we just viewed. In the Cosmos episode, they used the term *hologram* to describe a theoretical construct explaining a model of reality that is 100 percent supported by the complex mathematics used to describe our reality. This is a great way to conceptualize how the quantum fields work, but on the larger scale of the universe, as opposed to within the limited context of black holes.

When you think about how everything we see and are, is simply a perturbation in the various scalar fields, it makes a lot of sense to consider ourselves to be holograms, of sorts. The source of the information is unknown; but, this accurate description of ourselves, and everything else, as holograms derivative of the action of the quantum fields, rings true.

I like the assertion in the video that value is created by curating and organizing information in creative ways that are useful to others. Every byte of information in this book was always out there — it already existed — whether in my head, online, in other books, or out in the universe — but it already existed. As did the 26 letters of the alphabet I've organized in such a manner as to convey this information to you. Perhaps I synthesized a few *original* ideas, but what is that really?

There are some 55,000 words in this book, and 26 letters in the alphabet — ink molecules, paper molecules, ink and paper atoms, subatomic particles, fields (energy), and information conveyed to you in concert thereof. Any value herein lies in the organization of the information I sifted through and experiences I applied (also information encoded in my memory in the form of information), put together in such a way that it is useful to you. Ideas born of the fields, curated by a conscious being derivative of the fields (me), imparted via the fields (book/computer) to another conscious being comprised of the fields (you).

Which leads us to our next point: If the information contained in this book is simply *field information* that doesn't really *do* anything because we're all derivative of the exact same information or fields as the material in the book, then what exactly is being *done* when you read this material? Well, one thing that I believe is being done by asking that question is that we are exposing a fundamental truth about our humanity. A truth that a number of sources referenced in this book have alluded to — that our human state of being is a severely limiting state in relation to our true state of being, which is spiritual, or energy, in nature — pure awareness or consciousness.

SUMMARY

STAGE 1 RECOVERY — PREVENT RELAPSE

+ Identifying as a possessor of dual citizenship — far more energy than matter — and connecting to the Universe, creates a sense of peace and belonging previously not experienced (when we identified as strictly material beings subject to Newtonian cause-and-effect physics). This sense of connection and belonging to the Universe decreases stress, and thus makes us more resilient against relapse.

+ Understanding that we are extensions of a greater conscious-ness, and connected to everyone through the continuous fields that permeate all of us, helps us to overcome the feelings of lone-liness and isolation inherent to those in active addiction.

STAGE 2 RECOVERY — REGAIN AUTHENTICITY

+ In our authentic state, the fields enable us to mobilize the Uni-verse to realize the ideal reality in which our ideal self walks.

+ Assertion of our True Self provides the most effective link to our aspirational self and reality.
+ As we gain experience in asserting our authenticity, and receive positive feedback from the Universe, it becomes self-evident that our False Self undermines our progress. This realization drives us to assert our authenticity, gaining faith that by doing so, we are happier and life becomes effortless.

STAGE 3 RECOVERY — ENHANCE SPIRITUAL CAPACITY

+ The mathematics that governs the Universe must have an author.
+ Information is the most elemental, indivisible aspect of the Universe.
+ Information defines everything and everyone in the Universe.
+ As beings derivative of information, we are one with the Universe. Understanding this connects us with a higher power.
+ We are indivisible from a higher power.

CHAPTER 15

HOW CONSCIOUSNESS WORKS

Our consciousness is a unifying force — an ambassador with dual citizenship between the energy-based spiritual world and the material reality of daily experience, making us supernatural.

OUR PASSPORT TO DUAL CITIZENSHIP

Although we are all part of the same system, we are also differentiated from each other in some ways. I propose that it is our unique consciousness that accounts for this. Our consciousness is the *ghost in the machine* that makes me Me, and you You.

Our consciousness, our unique electromagnetic signature, is that pure state of awareness that Mooji says is timeless, and indestructible.

It is one aspect that distinguishes us from everyone else — yet, as energy and part of the quantum field — *connects* us to everyone else.

Consciousness is the immaterial half of our dual citizenship between the quantum and material worlds. It enables us to materialize our destiny and happiness by virtue of its mutual connection to the Universe, and our Higher Power.

The "Science & Non-Duality" website states the following:

> *Progress in theoretical physics during the past decade has led to a progressively more unified understanding of the laws of nature, culminating in the recent discovery of completely unified field theories based on the superstring. These theories identify a single universal, unified field at the basis of all forms and phenomena in the universe.*

> *At the same time, cutting-edge research in the field of neuroscience has revealed the existence of a 'unified field of consciousness'— a fourth major state of human consciousness, which is physiologically and subjectively distinct from waking, dreaming and deep sleep. In this meditative state, a.k.a. Samadhi, the threefold structure of waking experience — the observer, the observed and the process of observation — are united in one indivisible wholeness of pure consciousness.*

> *These parallel discoveries of a unified field of physics and a unified field of consciousness raise fundamental questions concerning the relationship between the two. We present compelling theoretical and experimental evidence that the unified field of physics and the unified field of consciousness are identical — i.e., that during the meditative state, human awareness directly experiences the unified field at the foundation of the universe . . . We briefly discuss mechanisms from quantum mechanics, quantum field theory, and superstring theory that could explain the proposed link between human neurophysiology and the unified field of physics.*

It is impossible to engage in any sort of communion with a Divine Intelligence without taking consciousness and the quantum field into account.

The following lecture by Dr. John Hagelin defines our consciousness as a bridge between material reality, and the Divine Intelligence — the quantum fields being the medium through which we commune.

 15.1

I have found that the state of awareness necessary to access the quantum fields — a pure state of consciousness — is most accessible by way of the teachings of Mooji. His guided meditations strip us of our identity in order to become something closer to a pure state of awareness — a state in which I may commune with a higher power.

Consciousness is pure energy with intent. We transmit our intent out into the field, and create the reality in which we choose to live.

Part of effective practice of UTR is shedding our identity — forgetting who we were — to become something more closely resembling a fully-realized version of ourselves. A quote in *Finding Joe* states that, "We must become willing to let go of the life that we had planned in order to have that which awaits us." Joe Dispenza states, "We cannot have a new personal reality as the same personality. We must literally become someone else." For those adopting the UTR change model, we *must* adopt the spiritual aspect of our personality to leverage the Universe.

One of my favorite modelers of dual citizenship is Ram Dass, whose documentary helps us appreciate the intrinsic value of adopting a more Eastern spiritual philosophy, and shedding the identity we have worked so hard to develop.

15.2

In becoming *no one*, we shed our earthly identity to commune with our Higher Power effectively. In doing so, we gain access to an unlimited source of love. Ram Dass would say that this source of love, our Higher Power, is an internal solution to the internal problems we hoped to resolve through our addictions.

HOW OUR HUMAN FORM IS LIMITING

The intent of the book is to catalyze change. If you and I are part and parcel of exactly the same information or field system, then in theory, we both already had access to this information — negating the necessity for me to compile and organize it into a book, or for you to internalize it and change.

Yet, presumably, you are reading this book because you do not possess the information presented. Why do we all NOT have all the information now? I would suggest it is because we are not presently in our ideal state of being. Our human state, or what Ram Dass likes to refer to as our *earth suit*, is severely limiting and imperfect when compared to our consciousness state — which he would say accounts for a majority of our frustration with both ourselves and each other.

Earnie Larsen observes how human imperfection impairs relationships in his book, *Believing in Myself,* when he states, ". . . how can any partner or friend be perfect? When we imagine that there will never be spaces in our togetherness, that there will always be complete agreement and fidelity, we set ourselves up for disappointment. *Even our friendship with God is limited by our own partial ability to be a friend.*" This passage highlights the discrepancy between our true, consciousness state of being and that which we embody in human form. Assuming God is perfect, then any shortcomings in our ability to love, or be loved by God, must come from *our* end of the equation — deficits wholly imposed by our limiting human state.

In our true, spiritual state of being, we are not separated from the Universe nor a higher power. We are pure awareness and consciousness, energy unconstrained by the limited, electrochemical cocktails that comprise the anger, sadness, or loneliness we experience in our earthly bodies. As consciousness, we are not limited by our five senses, because in a spiritual state, we don't need them.

In *Finding Joe*, the commentator conveying the Golden Buddha parable states that, ". . . we were born perfect, all-knowing, at one with God and the Universe . . ." — implying that it was only upon becoming human, and exposed to other imperfect humans, that we too became imperfect.

Gabor Mate' states that as children, when exposed to other imperfect beings, we began repressing our True Self. The discrepancy between our True Self, and the one that we publicly assert, became the root of all physical and mental pathology, including addiction.

So, in a meditative state we are able to shed many limiting aspects of our humanity, and as such, more closely identify with our true, spiritual state of being — a state of pure awareness, in which we may more closely identify with a higher power — in which we all *know* each other, we know all information, and above all, we know Love.

SUMMARY

STAGE 1 RECOVERY — PREVENT RELAPSE

+ Understanding that we hold dual citizenship between the material and immaterial world affords us hope and connection that decrease stress, particularly when in a meditative state.

+ Realizing that our identity is primarily spiritual in nature, we are able to put worldly problems into proper context, decreasing anxiety and relapse potential.

+ The more time we spend in our true state of being — a spiritual state — we realize the futility of the False Self, and begin to be less affected by others' opinions of us. This state of peace makes us more resilient against the stresses of our material, worldly self.

STAGE 2 RECOVERY — REGAIN AUTHENTICITY

+ As we gain depth of insight into our true nature, we begin to realize that our True Self is spiritual. Our authentic self is simply a reflection of what our Higher Power wishes most for us — to be happy and self-fulfilled, constantly growing, and having daily experiences filled with gratitude and love.

+ Recognizing the limitations of our *earth suit* provides context for understanding of our true, timeless, indestructible nature as a member of the Universe.

STAGE 3 RECOVERY — ENHANCE SPIRITUAL CAPACITY

+ When we understand that our True Self is spiritual in nature, spirituality becomes an inevitable aspect of both our self-perception and worldview.

+ Dual citizenship is temporary. Before we were born, and after we die, we revert to pure energy form having no further need for our limiting material state of being.

+ Grasping the limitations imposed on our True Self by overidentifying with the material world provides incentive to expand our experiences and understanding of the immaterial world.

CONCLUSION

A NEW UNDERSTANDING

The Unified Theory of Recovery change model may be applied with equal validity within the construct of any existing spiritual model — the fields serving as the instrument of any higher power. The *source* of information may be any higher power you choose to name. I personally prefer an ambiguous higher power; but, there is no discrepancy in plugging in your own deity as the fountainhead of all information.

In this model, an individual's consciousness — their timeless, formless state-of-being or Awareness — is not defined in relation to anything nor anyone in the material world. In pure awareness, neither time nor distance are relevant, thanks to the nature of quantum fields. There are no traditional boundaries on this plane of existence.

It is on this plane that we mutually "miss" each other, or "were just thinking of" each other. How many times have you gotten a text or call from someone who just happened to be on your mind a moment prior? This is the field at work between two citizens of the spiritual realm.

The field is continuous. It is everywhere, all of the time, simultaneously. You may be 3,000 miles away from a loved one with whom you have a connection — and from the field's perspective, you may as well be right next to them. There is comfort in the realization of this truth, particularly with loneliness being a primary relapse trigger. When I am feeling lonely, I reach out via text to friends. Ironically, the same fields upon which those electronic signals travel from my phone to theirs are the selfsame fields of which we are all a part. We are never really alone when we view our existence through the prism of quantum field reality. Meditation intensifies our sense of connectedness in the absence of direct means of communication.

THE CLINICAL BENEFITS OF ADOPTING A HIGHER POWER

By the same token that introduction of a higher power resolves many problems at the scientific edge of our understanding — doing so also helps resolve many clinical recovery-based problems. Addiction is, at its heart, a pathological effort to emotionally self-regulate uncomfortable emotions like anxiety, fear, shame, and anger, that stem from the meanings we assign to our circumstances.

Adopting a higher power such as that outlined in this book provides a tremendous shortcut toward overcoming addiction. Spending time in meditation, communing with a higher power, expedites our ability and willingness to adopt a spiritual perspective because of the experiential impact of such interventions. When we realize, through the academic teachings in this book, that we can leverage our meditational explorations to affect tangible outcomes, not only in ourselves, but also in our reality, the adoption of a spiritual perspective becomes even more compelling.

The UTR model's concept of a *benevolent* higher power is adopted from Eastern philosophies, and is devoid of the rules and regulations inherent to organized religion. This structure makes it so that traits such as low self-esteem, or spiritual contempt are not barriers to our ability to participate, because we are not being judged nor held in contempt.

Perhaps most importantly, a loving, benevolent higher power is intuitively attractive because we have often spent decades starving for unconditional love. Such a higher power provides a divine template with which to align our True Self and connect — beautifully.

The following concepts are crucial to the recovery process, and are *qualitative*, or subjective — much more closely related to the spiritual vs. the material realm:

- **Authenticity** — critical to human and spiritual connection
- **Honesty** — critical to self-esteem and relational dynamics
- **Values** — living in integrity with defined values yields happiness
- **Aspiration** — regain hope and purpose
- **Hope** — quantum uncertainty promotes quick change
- **Love** — connection with a benevolent higher power
- **Congruence** — between head and heart — confidence
- **Connection** — with multiple sources of love
- **Trust** — that "everything is as it should be"
- **Gut Instincts** — ability to navigate social situations
- **Fearlessness** — reveling in the unknown (vs. anxiety)
- **Happiness** — living with purpose and integrity
- **Self-Awareness** — conscious observer (vs. victim of our thoughts)
- **Growth** — unlimited potential and possibility

- **Congruence** — creates electromagnetic quantum coherence and trust
- **Consistency** — authentic identity does not change
- **Self-Esteem** — restored with assertion of authenticity
- **Trust** — in a higher power, in gut instincts, and in others — interdependence

Because those with a spiritual bent usually assign stronger meaning to them than would a skeptic, and therapy is about using words to elicit emotions to catalyze change, working on these subjective concepts will have far less emotional impact on skeptics than those with a spiritual identity.

So, skepticism vs. spirituality is not a moral argument. It is a clinical argument that enables us to choose between an anemic quality of recovery vs. an enhanced depth, rate, scope, and longevity of recovery.

The idea that, by going the spiritual route we get to become co-gods, creating our ideal selves and reality in the process, turns out to be just a bonus.

The extent to which I have been able to integrate field-based spirituality into my worldview is the extent to which I have made gains in the above areas, resulting in increased resilience, confidence, self-respect, and more fulfilling relationships. The emotional benefits have outweighed any philosophical reservations I may have had about adopting such a perspective, which, if you think of it, is the whole idea behind faith.

I make no *epistemological* claims for the existence of God. This is impossible anyway, because it is not possible to make objective claims as a subjective part of any closed system. Again, there is a reason they call it faith.

UTR, as with any recovery program, is ultimately about *doing*. I encourage all patients to engage in *doing* traditional Stage One and Stage Two recovery activities to supplement our work, including *attending* regular mutual support groups, *developing* a sober support network, and *reading* recovery-based materials.

The maintenance aspect of UTR — meditation — is addictive in itself. The more it is done, the more we want to do it. Initially I was skeptical about whether meditation would yield any benefits. But the more I was exposed to quality-guided meditations, the more I felt compelled to do them. The more I did, the more feedback from the Universe I got in the form of synchronicities validating my efforts.

Even now, when asked to elaborate on this aspect of my spiritual practice, I pull back a little bit because I know how I used to reflexively shut down when other people would discuss their spirituality. UTR's brand of spirituality is a very personal thing. As such, I am extremely conscious of appearing to judge anyone for not subscribing to my own personal brand. I know what it is like to sit next to a spiritual zealot on an airplane or in a social setting and feel judged for not endorsing whatever model they're passionate about.

UTR spirituality is intentionally ambiguous. It is completely self-oriented. There is no *right* way to do it. My personal practices undoubtedly will differ from others' because some meditations, for example, work for us while others don't. Other practitioners may embrace techniques that don't resonate with me. The details are less important than the overriding principles. Everyone's vision for their idealized self and reality are unique.

What is important is that those who have integrated UTR have rapidly gained the therapeutic benefits of faith in a higher power, which include:

- peace of mind,
- peace of heart,
- confidence,
- a resource to combat loneliness,
- decreased anxiety from worrying about outcomes,
- increased self-efficacy,
- relief in the knowledge that they don't have to do everything themselves,
- connection to an unlimited source of love, and
- a sense of acceptance by the Universe of their True Self (which contrasts with how the higher power of their childhood might have accepted them).

Many patients have related that engagement in guided meditations was akin to taking a substance — a peaceful state devoid from the environmental stressors of the day. Meditational formats serve different purposes; and some I prefer over others, and for different reasons. For instance, for shedding worldly awareness and getting my connection on with the Universe, Mooji's a great way to go. With his meditations, I am able to *become no one*, which is a wonderful state. He has hundreds of free guided meditations on YouTube, as well as numerous paid distribution outlets including Tidal and Amazon Prime.

The following is an example of one of Mooji's shorter YouTube guided meditations:

 16.1

Communing with a higher power helps us accomplish many things beneficial to recovery, including: decreasing our overall stress level, dissociating from environmental stressors, and increasing our faith. In a meditative state of "mindlessness" we begin mobilizing the Universe. We take advantage of its *goodness*, and benefit from its desire for us to be happy and fulfill our potential.

It is also in this state where we gain more experience *becoming no one*. Our worldly identity serves as a limiting factor; so, we must learn to *forget* our residual self-image on a daily basis.

Through practice (*doing*), meditation solves two problems inherent to early recovery from addiction — spiritual contempt and lack of hope (low self-efficacy). In a meditative state, with our heads and hearts congruently aligned, we allow the Universe to conspire in our favor, compressing the time between now and when our aspirations are realized. More importantly, we become *happy* in the process.

PROMISES KEPT

The AA Big Book has something that many in the program are familiar with — The Promises of Alcoholics Anonymous. Prior to beginning this UTR journey, I was frustrated at my inability to strongly identify with them. But *all* came true as I fully integrated, and internalized, the principles outlined in this book:

Promise 1: *We are going to know a new freedom and a new happiness*

Promise 2: *We will not regret the past nor wish to shut the door on it.*

Promise 3: *We will comprehend the word serenity.*

Promise 4: *We will know peace.*

Promise 5: *No matter how far down the scale we have gone, we will see how our experience can benefit others.*

Promise 6: *The feeling of uselessness and self-pity will disappear.*

Promise 7: *We will lose interest in selfish things and gain interest in our fellows.*

Promise 8: *Self-seeking will slip away.*

Promise 9: *Our whole attitude and outlook upon life will change.*

Promise 10: *Fear of people and economic insecurity will leave us.*

Promise 11: *We will intuitively know how to handle situations which used to baffle us.*

Promise 12: *We will suddenly realize that God is doing for us what we could not do for ourselves.*

The Promises began coming into fruition for me *somewhat* before I mastered UTR principles; but, it was only after engaging in UTR that I was able to strongly relate to every one of these promises. They have all come true, and now hold more meaning for me than ever before. This is one of the gifts of recovery with a spiritual bent.

The purpose of this book, as previously stated, is three-fold:

1. To make a plausible argument to those in addiction or recovery that their past has nothing to do with their future,

2. That there is a benevolent higher power that *wants*, above all, for them to fully realize their full potential, and

3. That the mechanisms by which we may accomplish this exist in the quantum field.

With the true nature of reality clearly defined and proven, and our ability to materially affect reality through the use of consciousness proven experimentally *and* experientially, the table is now set for you to engage in quantum change with full confidence. We can, without doubt, leverage the principles outlined in this book to design a future of our own creation in conspiracy with a higher power who permeates the *entire* system to the benefit of ourselves and of those we love.

In applying the principles outlined in UTR, we transform from being spiritually challenged to becoming individuals who possess and assert our dual citizenship status with confidence. We unify the material and immaterial worlds, and select a more compelling reality from the *infinite* number of possible realities — a life path where addiction is replaced by joy, fulfillment, and gratitude.

We have seen how our present actions affect both our future *and* our past. We know that an idealized vision of ourselves serves as a beacon on the horizon toward which we must move, defined by new, and sometimes old, consciously-chosen values. We leverage the quantum field, and our relationship with the Universe, to expedite our journey to this new reality — compressing the time between now and then — where the predominant emotion is gratitude. The effortlessness of our journey becomes the measure of our spiritual progress.

It is impossible to adequately comprehend the nature of reality in the absence of a spiritual perspective.

THE UTR CONCEPTION OF THE NATURE OF THE UNIVERSE IS AS FOLLOWS:

- The Universe is not static, but dynamic — possessing a consciousness.
- The Universe is inherently benevolent — it wants good.
- We ourselves, and everything, are indivisible from the quantum field.

- The quantum field is a two-way vehicle through which we both commune with, and receive feedback from, the Universe.
- All conscious beings are connected through the field.
- The quantum field represents infinite possibilities at any given point in time.
- We each author our own realities, either consciously or unconsciously, by selecting from an infinite number of possibilities, every moment.
- The richness of an idealized (future) vision of ourselves and our world, along with the frequency, quality, and coherence of our meditational efforts, dictates the quality of feedback reciprocated by the Universe.
- There is no one-way "arrow of time." What we perceive as future aspirations are "future memories" corresponding to an idealized state of being, which exists in one potential reality serving as a beacon toward which we may direct our energies — vs. siphoning them off in the form of fruitless distractions (such as addiction).
- The Universe "wants" us to be happy, walking in a reality akin to our own version or definition of Heaven on Earth where gratitude is the predominant emotion, and in which our potential is fully realized.
- Living in our absolutely most-authentic state in the present affords us the best opportunity to realize the reality in which we aspire to walk — compressing the time between now and then.

The material in this book, and the sources from which it came, make it difficult to refute these tenets.

The predominant moral imperative among nearly all religions and spiritual philosophies is to become the best possible version of ourselves. It is in this state that we are happiest, and filled with gratitude. In such a state we are not inclined to self-medicate. It's that simple. The ancient Eastern philosophers intuitively knew this, and it still holds true today.

BUT WHAT ABOUT YOU?!

Many ask whether I have realized my own idealized state of existence. My response is always, "Not yet." I also point out that:

1. If you'll recall, the point of the *Magic Wand Thought Experiment* is to generate an aspirational ideal to move toward. As I underwent the changes outlined in this book, I became consistently more content and comfortable in my shoes. Realizing the ultimate vision is not necessary to provide a remarkable degree of relief from stress. That is not to say that I do not continue to aspire toward an ideal; it simply means that we do not have to get all the way there in order for this program to work.

2. My idealized future vision is a moving target, as is everyone's vision who undergoes the UTR process. This is for many reasons:

   a. We shift our focus as we get to know ourselves better, particularly early-on in the process.

   b. As we realize that this actually works, we also start realizing that we were likely thinking too small, and thus increase our vision to something more accurately reflective of what we now believe is possible.

   c. As we grow, we may decide to move in another direction.

Western religions have a sort of *collective* vision of what is accept-able and necessary to "succeed" on *their* terms. UTR is a more self-oriented, or perhaps *self-full,* and intimate spiritual model. Why not experience heaven on earth *now* vs. waiting until we're dead to experience it?

Our greatest *state of happiness* is when we are in the *process* of realizing, and growing into, our true potential. I suspect that once we have arrived at that *state of being* we will find new aspirations, inspired by the fact that we have come so far. Why stop, right?

Once you have internalized this material, you will want to see how far you can take your recovery. You will identify less as an addict, and more as a person who used to suffer from addiction, and who considers your experiences in addiction as a necessary, and valuable, part of your life. You will take pride in having overcome a disease that many succumb to, becoming an inspiration to others that they, too, might put the Universe to work for themselves.

THE 12 STEPS AND UTR

Twelve-Step programs and the Unified Theory of Recovery (UTR) are both change models and their objectives are aligned with each other. They provide a construct by which individuals may move from active addiction to freedom from addiction, becoming capable of engaging in healthy relationships.

Approximately 10 percent of the U.S. population could be clinically diagnosed with some sort of substance-use disorder on any given day. The average American has a social footprint — family, friends, co-workers, etc. — of about 10 people, so it would be reasonable to posit that everyone in the U.S. either knows or is an addict. And that is just substances.

Many have what we call *process addictions*. As the name implies, people with a process addiction engage in behavior that negatively impacts primary relationships, or functionality in a dimension such as work, school, home upkeep, time management, finances, physical, emotional, recreational, or social interactions. Examples of process addictions include gambling, spending, shopping, gaming, porn, sex itself, relationships, food, TV, etc. If you combine substance use disorders and behavioral addictions, that number easily exceeds 10 percent of the population.

Addiction is the #1 public health crisis in the country at this time and is also the least-funded public health area by a substantial margin, largely due to social stigma.

There are many ways to recover from addiction, but the most common is the 12-Step Program identified with Alcoholics Anonymous, developed during the 1930s in the United States.

UTR dovetails nicely with the core tenets of the 12 Steps, and I always encourage patients to attend 12-Step meetings or some other mutual support group to supplement their UTR work. There are many reasons for this, not the least of which is the necessity for those in recovery to develop a mutual support system consisting of others in recovery. Boredom and loneliness are the top two culprits in relapse, and the fellowship afforded those in the recovery community is indispensable for one's long-term prospects. UTR is at its early stages — as was AA at one point (consisting of just two individuals: Dr. Bob and Bill W.) — so presently, there is no worldwide fellowship of UTR practitioners — although I expect that number to increase; and, a community-like web page will be established to facilitate this vision.

The principles of UTR correlate with the 12 Steps in many ways. Let us now go through the twelve steps in order, and see how the two models are complementary.

1. We admitted we were powerless over alcohol — that our lives had become unmanageable.

UTR says that acknowledging our past is important, if only to leverage it to drive us forward, *away* from old habits and their consequences. We have, in fact, been powerless to stop our addictions in the past, or there would be no need to change; but, past performance does not guarantee future results. So, UTR substitutes power where there once was powerlessness by harnessing the dynamics of the quantum field whereby we select our reality via communion with our Higher Power.

2. Came to believe that a Power greater than ourselves could restore us to sanity.

UTR addresses the core issues of those who struggle with the idea of a higher power. One problem for many entering recovery from active addiction relates to their past conceptions of a higher power. They bring issues of trust, resentment, fear, and what is referred to in my line of work as the "righting reflex" — the idea that we do not like being told what to do — into recovery, creating resistance to adoption of a world view containing spirituality.

One reason that many in recovery have aversion to authority figures stems from the childhood relationship they had with dysfunctional parents who represented the closest thing to a God that existed. Their parents were neglectful, addicted, and prone to bouts of anger and rage; yet, they were dragged to church every week — not understanding the hypocrisy between the parents the Bible told them they should have, and that which they experienced on a daily basis.

Children do not have the scope of perspective adults have, so by default, they assign the dysfunctional attributes displayed by their all-powerful parents to God, coming to conclusions about God based upon that experience. As a result not only do they not trust God, but because of their incredibly low self-esteem they wonder how any God would want anything to do with them. That was before substances got ahold of them. This sentiment only increased as their addictions took hold and their disease progressed. As such, belief in a benevolent higher power — much less one who would consider them worthy of restoration to sanity — is often a huge disconnect.

It is no wonder many have trouble with the spiritual aspects of the 12 Steps. With UTR, there is a much more loosely-defined higher power — one which has for us two prime directives: to become the best possible version of ourselves, and to be as happy as possible. UTR affords us the means by which to employ the quantum field — and therefore the Universe — to this end. With UTR, we partner with our Higher Power to affect change toward the kind of sanity that recovery of our True Self provides.

3. Made a decision to turn our will and our lives over to the care of God as we understood God.

UTR makes this step easier than traditional Western spiritual conceptions do for the same reasons it makes Step 2 easier. With UTR, it is easier to trust, and therefore "turn our will and our lives over" primarily because it is we who define the will of our Higher Power — to become the most fully-realized version of ourselves. We get to define the values that *we* see as best supporting *our* vision for *our* most realized and happiest version of ourselves, which is the will of our Higher Power for *our* lives. There are no demands, rules, judgments, nor threats to activate our righting reflex — only a sense that if we hoist our sails, we will harness the benevolent wind of the Universe, which will draw us toward the ideal self and reality of our own design. Perhaps our innate aspirations were instilled by our Higher Power? If so, we are doing Its will.

4. Made a searching and fearless moral inventory of ourselves.

UTR aligns with Step 4 when we clearly define not only our idealized future vision for ourselves, but also, when we consciously identify aspects of our personality we wish to discard — those unhelpful in moving us toward our designed future self or reality. This step is critical in both change models. We may wish to use the AA Big Book, Step 4 template, to help identify those character defects we wish to shed.

5. Admitted to God, to ourselves, and to another human being the exact nature of our wrongs.

Step 5 aligns with UTR in that we benefit by shedding behaviors with which we will no longer identify — lying, cheating, stealing, duplicity, etc. Sharing these aspects with another person is a cleansing experience, delineating that which is behind us, from that which is in front of us. It is ejecting the garbage and baggage from our past, lightening our burden moving forward, and making change easier. This makes us nimbler in our journey toward our idealized future reality.

6. We were entirely ready to have God remove all these defects of character.

Step 6 is completely in alignment with the UTR process of aligning ourselves with the Universe. We are living daily in a manner that most closely resembles our idealized future self through daily guided meditation. Through this process we bring back, from our meditative state, characteristics our idealized self possesses. This process necessarily replaces past defects of character.

7. Humbly asked God to remove our shortcomings.

Step 7 is done in the UTR meditation process or experience. No shortcomings exist in our meditative state of pure awareness where we *become no one*. The more time spent in this state, the closer we commune with the Universe or our Higher Power who removes our shortcomings.

8. Made a list of all persons we had harmed and became willing to make amends to them all.

The 12 Steps and UTR approach this in different ways; but, practitioners of both modes of recovery agree that the best way to make amends is to become the best possible version of ourselves. Walking in integrity is called, *living amends*. UTR practitioners have no problem with making amends by conventional means.

9. Made direct amends to such people wherever possible, except when to do so would injure them or others.

The way that most people make amends to others, other than materially, is by being different from the person they were when in active addiction. Nearly all report that those to whom they make amends tend to say essentially the same thing, "The best way you can make amends to me is to continue on the path you're on as a changed person." If financial amends are in order, it is only in the state of recovery where we will become able to develop the financial means to make those amends.

Those who were harmed in some other way never want to experience the same pain that we imposed upon them while we were a past version of ourselves. Increasing our growth toward our idealized self is the amend that keeps on giving.

10. Continued to take personal inventory and when we were wrong promptly admitted it.

Quality recovery, whether 12 Step or UTR, requires continuity over an extended time frame — preferably indefinitely. Step 10 is to be used daily. Daily UTR guided meditations prompt us to reflect upon the day to assess where we have fallen short of being our idealized, fully-realized self. There is consistency between these programs, as daily reflection on our progress, and adherence-to, recovery principles maximizes our potential for long-term success.

11. Sought through prayer and meditation to improve our conscious contact with God, as we understood Him, praying only for knowledge of His will for us and the power to carry that out.

Meditation is UTR's form of prayer, and so, is in alignment with Step 11. A tenet of UTR is communing as often as possible, through meditation, with the Universe. We put out a congruent vision for our idealized self and reality while in a meditative state of pure awareness. It is in this state we can experience insights from divine intelligence — via the quantum field — that informs our daily existence when we are *not* in a meditative state. With UTR, we are able to employ the Universe to facilitate the realization of our divine vision.

Our Higher Power conspires to make living effortless — decreasing stress and infusing us with a confidence and warmth unavailable to those not engaged in this level of spirituality. The Universe's will for us is not a mystery. It is to recover our True and Authentic self, and to assert that authenticity while striving to realize our potential. Our vision is likely to shift as we evolve; and often at the beginning of the practice, we realize that we were thinking too small. Noticing this is part of the process. *Progress, not perfection* is not a slogan that is unique to AA.

12. Having had a spiritual awakening as the result of these Steps, we tried to carry this message to alcoholics, and to practice these principles in all our affairs.

Step 12 and UTR are aligned because it is impossible to live a UTR lifestyle without attracting those drawn to our Zen-like, non-reactivity, and the confidence with which we navigate the unknown. With UTR, we become *walking* "12th-Steps," both internally and externally.

The 12 Steps and UTR are partners in recovery.

ACKNOWLEDGMENTS

I wish to thank those whose knowing or unknowing contributions were essential to my ability to have written this book (and in no particular order).

My wife Linda, who tolerated my long hours as I worked two jobs.

My son Nick, who weathered my addictions and still talks to me. My daughter Heather, who weathered my addictions and doesn't, but who as a result, taught me that environmental factors mustn't dictate our happiness.

My parents Dudley W. and Mary C. Pierce, who did what parents do. My brother David, who always provides an alternative perspective. My sister Melissa, because if I don't mention her, I'll never hear the end of it.

Jimmy Weiss and Steven Tyler, for keeping me from leaving Betty Ford on Day 1. Michael Potter, my counselor at Betty Ford, for being so good at what he does, and for reviewing my manuscript.

John Henderlite, my counselor at age 17, and my friend and colleague today — and fellow bass player — and his wife, Cindy. John Easton (R.I.P.) — my counselor back in the day whose sage advice included, "Knock it off."

Dan Frigo, Ph.D., for his ongoing moral, academic, and psychological support throughout this project — and the cigar. Casey Portner, for hiring me fresh out of grad school, being a friend and colleague, and for contributing to many ideas touched on in this book. The Keller Family, for providing the breathing room, time, and the facility in which to incubate the ideas that became this book.

All of my exes, past, present, and future (see what I did there?).

Captain Morgan, absinthe, the letter D, and various cartels.

Jason Kays, who knows way too much about me, and who actually *read* the early manuscript and provided useful feedback. Ed DeFour, Jeff Borgeson, Nate Latta — the band — who facilitated my field research leading up to the project.

My editor, Heather Davis Desrocher, and publisher, April O'Leary.

William Kyle Malott, who years ago gave me a job when there were none.

The faculty and administration of The Hazelden Betty Ford Graduate School of Addiction Studies.

My ACA home group members. My clinical colleagues at Counseling of Southwest Florida.

Whomever drove me to Betty Ford that one day.

ALL of my patients — past, present, and future.

ABOUT
THE AUTHOR

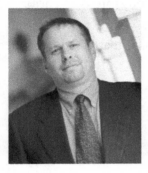 Andrew Pierce is a person in long-term recovery from multiple addictions.

Adopted as an infant, he was diagnosed with childhood (and later, adult) ADD. Andrew began using recreational drugs and alcohol at age 13, and continued use through age 17 when, following some legal issues, he was compelled to attend treatment and then a sober living stint in the Twin Cities (Minneapolis-St. Paul, MN).

Following that treatment episode, he remained abstinent from substances for 13 years until relapsing on his 30th birthday when he gave himself permission to have, "a nice glass of wine" that led to an 18-year relapse during which he lost everything; his business, family, two wives, and nearly his life on many occasions.

On April 26th of 2014, he entered treatment at The Betty Ford Center in Rancho Mirage, CA, and has since been in continuous recovery.

Andrew is a graduate of the Hazelden Betty Ford Graduate School of Addiction Studies, having had the honor of being the second student in school history to be allowed to lecture to the entire patient population.

He possesses the highest addiction credential available in the state of Florida, the MCAP (Master's Certification for Addiction Professionals), and is currently in private practice at Counseling of Southwest Florida in Naples, FL (www.counselingswfl.com) where he works with those in, or recovering from, addiction as well as co-occurring mental health disorders in order to help them fulfill their true potential.

Andrew crafted the Unified Theory of Recovery (UTR) clinical model to benefit patients who have difficulty with the spiritual aspect of recovery due to his own inability to buy into conventional spiritual paradigms. He has had great success implementing this clinical model, and will be authoring additional material to enable other clinicians to bring the UTR clinical model to addiction treatment settings throughout the world.

CPSIA information can be obtained
at www.ICGtesting.com
Printed in the USA
LVHW111057260123
737493LV00001B/6